Recognizing Botulism

New Insights from Old Narratives

Medical Narratives on
120 People with Botulism
1902-1931

J.A. Talkington, PhD

Cherity Cook, Editor

Makenzie Eldridge, Research Assistant

DEDICATIONS

Ruby Lynch
(1895-1913)
Student, Stanford University
Her death sparked funding for botulism research.

Georgina (Brackenridge) Spooner Burke
(1886-1960)
Education at Vassar and Columbia was funded
by George Brackenridge, a family friend.
Research Scientist at Stanford University
With courage, she boldly exposed how corporate
funding had compromised the integrity of
academic research meant to inform the public
about food safety.

Murray Sales
(1865-1951)

```
"It is not because I expect ever again to
be afflicted personally in that way, but
for the sake of humanity and for others,
I am determined to do all in my power to
lessen the fatalities caused by those who
think less of human life than of
profits." - Murray Sales 2/13/1921
```

As a father of children poisoned by botulinum toxin,
he showed what one voice could accomplish in
advocating for consumer safety.

Friends, family, and colleagues patiently
indulged my endless stories about botulism
research. I am so grateful for all the
encouragement and criticism. Only my mother
believed I would finish this book; she was right.

CONTENTS

RECOGNIZING BOTULISM

CONTENTS CONTAINING TOXIN

ACKNOWLEDGMENTS

I am deeply grateful to the historical societies and to the descendants of those victims featured in this book. Your ancestors have become like my own, and I am honored to share their stories. It is my hope that this work honors the memory of those who tragically lost their lives to botulism.

Thank you to all of the proofreaders.

To the dozens of researchers and physicians who practiced medicine in the era that advanced the understanding of botulism, appreciation goes to:

Dr. Robert Allen	Dr. George Armstrong
Dr. J.A. Belanger	Dr. Stanley Black
Dr. William Carey	Dr. Culbertson
Dr. J.P. Dewitt	Dr. E.C. Dickson
Dr. Herb Emmerson	Dr. J.C. Geiger
Dr. J.A.R. Glancy	Dr. Robert Graham
Dr. Hoover	Dr. Emil Otto Jellinek
Dr. C.G. Jennings	Dr. Frank L. Kelly
Dr. LaChapelle	Dr. W.H. Long
Dr. L.F. Mutschmann	Dr. John Phillips
Dr. John G. Spencer	Dr. H.C. Watkins
Dr. Ray Wilbur	Dr. William Mayo
Dr. Charles Mayo	Dr. A.R. McMahon
Dr. E.J. McConnell	Dr. William Ophuls
Dr. C.A. Poage	Dr. Polk
Dr. W.T. Rathburn	Dr. John Roach
Dr. Chris Sheppard	Dr. Donald R. Smith
Dr. W.R. Witwer	Dr. Weigandt
Dr. A.A. Whittemore	Dr. E.H. French
Dr. Eugene Johnson	Dr. Alpheus Jennings
Dr. Victor C Vaughan	

As the author, I have made every effort to ensure the accuracy and completeness of the information presented in this book. However, I make no representations or warranties regarding the accuracy, completeness, or reliability of the content. Any errors or omissions are entirely my own, and I assume full responsibility for any inaccuracies or mistakes. The views expressed in this book are mine and do not necessarily reflect the opinions of any organizations or institutions mentioned.

I welcome correspondence with the descendants of the people in this book or other botulism historians if any exist. The email for the book is:

RecognizingBotulism@gmail.com

Hopefully, more details and photographs will come my way, allowing me to update this manuscript with a new version of *Recognizing Botulism.*

RECOGNIZING BOTULISM

RECOGNIZING BOTULISM

How Death Came, Unbidden, to Mrs. Sales' Dinner Party

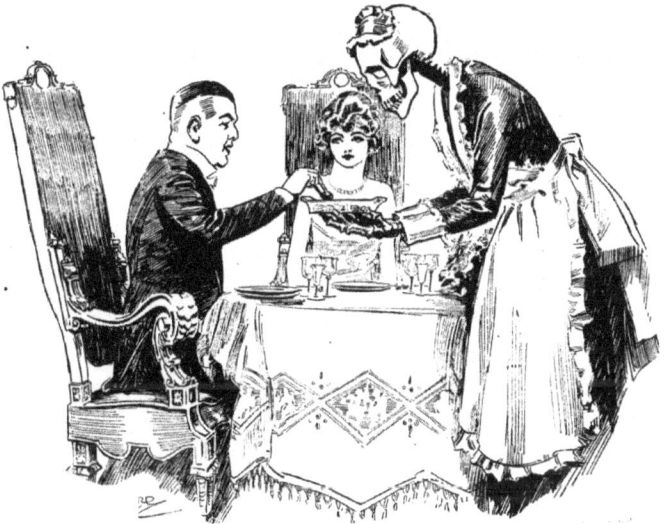

A graphic from a newspaper in 1919 depicting the
maid serving Murray Sales canned ripe olives.

RECOGNIZING BOTULISM

PREFACE

The Inspiration

The inspiration for this book stems from remaining curious about a research conundrum I encountered while studying historical botulism. In modern medicine, the *initial* misdiagnosis rate for botulism is very high. But that wasn't always the case. Physicians in the early 1900s became quite adept at diagnosing botulism, even though most had no firsthand experience with botulism. How, I pondered for years, could that diagnostic skill be developed then lost to time?

I was fortunate to cross paths with Anna Ziede, PhD, at Oklahoma State University. She is the author of *Canned: The Rise and Fall of Consumer Confidence in the American Food Industry.* She shared the archival materials from the Stanford library unlocking many mysteries for me.

My father mentored me in genealogy during his latter years. This was how I was able to contact the descendants. My mother valued history. She maintained the family heirlooms in our family home as a constant reminder that the past has value.

Gratitude is also due to Peter Hall, PhD, from the Department of Government at Harvard University. Years ago, Dr. Hall accepted a phone call from me, a total stranger. He generously listened to my methodology challenges and then thoughtfully introduced me to a historical research methodology known as 'process tracing'. I honed this technique during my doctoral thesis. For this book, 'process tracing' enabled me to triangulate historical data, drawing on newspapers and vintage medical reports. This integration created a multifaceted narrative on botulism symptoms in historical outbreaks.

Diagnostic Challenges

A timely diagnosis is critical for effective treatment with the botulism antitoxin, yet research indicates that most cases of botulism are *initially* misdiagnosed. The chances of an accurate diagnosis improve when victims of a botulism outbreak present together, as part of a group, rather than as isolated cases. Botulism often mimics other conditions, each of which must be tested and ruled out before the correct diagnosis is made. As a result, botulism is often described as a "diagnosis of exclusion."

For many physicians, their understanding of botulism is based largely on medical textbooks that focus on the most severe forms of the disease. Mild botulism symptoms, however, are rarely addressed in the literature. Few physicians have encountered an actual case of foodborne botulism, and the decision to administer the botulism antitoxin depends on diagnosing botulism through clinically observable symptoms. Given the urgency of the situation, there is simply no time to wait for the results of laboratory tests from the Centers for Disease Control and Prevention.

History Informing the Present

As I delved into historical case studies published in medical journals from a century ago, I was struck by insights that, though still highly relevant, had been largely forgotten over time. One of the most significant revelations was the identification of atypical symptoms of botulism, which often lead to misdiagnosis. I discovered cases of asymmetrical paralysis and uneven muscle weakness in botulism victims, as well as instances of seizures, suggesting that the botulinum toxin penetrated into the brain. These findings offer valuable clues that could enhance the understanding and detection of botulism today.

In 1913, Dr. E.C. Dickson of Stanford University discovered brain lesions during an autopsy of a botulism victim. A few years later, he conducted an experiment in which he ground up human brain matter from another botulism fatality and fed it to a guinea pig, which subsequently developed botulism and died. This compelling evidence confirmed the toxin's ability to infiltrate the brain.

The benefit of a century's worth of hindsight proved invaluable, allowing me to reexamine hundreds of cases of foodborne botulism, uncovering critical patterns that warranted deeper investigation.

Science Primer

Botulism is caused by poisoning from botulinum toxin, which is produced by a spore-forming bacterium called *Clostridium botulinum*. This bacterium is commonly found in soil. Short answer: the disease develops in stages: first, the bacterium produces the toxin and then the toxin causes the disease of botulism.

Longer answer: When the bacterium grows in low-oxygen environments, such as improperly canned food, it releases botulinum toxin. Sometimes, the canned food container may swell; sometimes it won't. The food may also be in a state of decomposition, but botulinum toxin itself has no taste and no smell. Once botulinum toxin enters the bloodstream, it blocks acetylcholine release at neuromuscular junction, leading to flaccid paralysis. Flaccid means limp. Fatalities from botulism typically occur due to respiratory failure or a cardiac event.

In the early 1900s, foodborne botulism was the only type of botulism recognized. In the 1920s, researchers determined humans were susceptible to two strains: Type A and Type B, both causing foodborne botulism. Later, another strain, Type E, in fish was discovered to be toxic to humans. Currently, Types A-G have been identified.

There are five forms of human botulism:

- **foodborne** botulism
- **wound** botulism
- **adult intestinal** toxemia
- **infant** botulism (intestinal colonization from consuming spores orally)
- **inhalation** botulism (lab accident or biological war attack)
- **iatrogenic** botulism from pharmaceutical injections of botulinum toxin

Botulism is a challenging "diagnosis of exclusion," meaning that other conditions with similar symptoms must be ruled out. These include, but are not limited to, the following: Myasthenia Gravis, Guillain-Barré Syndrome, Lambert-Eaton Myasthenic Syndrome, Multiple Sclerosis, Tick Paralysis, Stroke or Transient Ischemic Attack, Organophosphate Poisoning, Pesticide or Food Poisoning, Diphtheria, Influenza, and Polio. Botulism has even been mistaken for drunkenness and mental health disorders.

Stages of Botulism

Medical education traditionally focuses on severe cases of foodborne botulism, where symptoms progress rapidly and dramatically. However, research shows that botulism manifests across a spectrum of severity, and this continuum is crucial for early diagnosis, especially in cases where symptoms may not be immediately severe or obvious. Based on the nuances I found in my research, I propose this general scale as a starting point to understand the range of impact.

1. **No botulism**
2. **Subclinical damage from botulism**
3. **Barely observable botulism**
4. **Mild botulism**
5. **Moderate botulism**
6. **Moderately severe botulism**
7. **Severe botulism**
8. **Life-threatening botulism (hospitalization required)**
9. **Permanent lifelong debilitating botulism**
10. **Fatal botulism**

Recognizing Botulism offers an in-depth exploration of the symptoms of untreated botulism, set in an era before the advent of antitoxin treatment. Written with scholarly rigor, this book establishes itself as a significant contribution to the history of science, offering new insights that deserve a place in the ongoing study of this dangerous and often misunderstood disease.

A Unique Contribution

There has never been a book quite like this on botulism, which is why I felt compelled to write a historically-accurate medical narrative that would be educational to the medical community and also be accessible (and interesting) to the general public. By illuminating the complexities of botulism, my hope is that this book will serve as a valuable resource—one that not only informs but also has the potential to save lives.

J.A. Talkington, PhD
RecognizingBotulism@gmail.com

Further reading for scholars and medical personnel:

For a complete study on this topic, read the medical articles cited in *Recognizing Botulism*.

Allen, Robert W., and A. Walter Ecklund. "Botulism in North Dakota: Report of Outbreak of Thirteen Fatal Cases." *Journal of the American Medical Association*, vol. 99, no. 7, 1932, pp. 557-559.

Armstrong, Charles. "Botulism from Eating Canned Ripe Olives." *Journal of Medical Research*, 1919. Free PDF download on Google Scholar

Black, Stanley. "Pathology of Ptomaine Poisoning." *Southern California Practitioner*, vol. 22, 1907
Found in HathiTrust.org

Kelly, Frank. California State Board of Health. "Investigation of Five Cases of Botulinus Poisoning at Colusa September 30, 1919." *California State Board of Health Report*, vol. 15, no. 4, 1919, p. 114.

Dickson, E. C. Botulism: A Clinical and Experimental Study. 1918.

Emerson, Herbert W., and George W. Collins. "Botulism from Canned Ripe Olives." *Journal of Laboratory and Clinical Medicine*, vol. 5, 1920, pp. 559-565.

Geiger, J. C. "An Outbreak of Botulism at St. Anthony's Hospital, Oakland, Calif., October, 1920." *Public Health Reports*, 1920, pp. 2858-2860.

Glancy, James Albert Ray. "Botulism–A Clinical Study of an Outbreak in the Yukon." *Canadian Medical Association Journal*, vol. 10, no. 11, 1920, p. 1027. Free PDF download from the National Institutes of Health, National Library of Medicine.

Jellinek, E. O. "Ptomaine Poisoning." *California State Journal of Medicine*, vol. 1, no. 4, 1903, p. 121. A free PDF download from NIH found through Google Scholar.

Jennings, C. G., et al. "An Outbreak of Botulism: Report of Cases." *Journal of the American Medical Association*, vol. 74, no. 2, 1920, pp. 77-80.

Lamanna, Carl. "The Most Poisonous Poison: What Do We Know About the Toxin of Botulism? What Are the Problems to Be Solved?" *Science*, vol. 130, no. 3378, 1959, pp. 763-772.

Tacket, Carol O., et al. "Equine Antitoxin Use and Other Factors That Predict Outcome in type A Foodborne Botulism." *The American Journal of Medicine*, vol. 76, no. 5, 1984, pp. 794-798.

ST Louis, Michael E., et al. "Botulism from chopped garlic: delayed recognition of a major outbreak." *Annals of Internal Medicine* 108.3 (1988): 363-368.

Sisco, Dwight L. "An outbreak of botulism." *Journal of the American Medical Association* 74.8 (1920): 516-521.

Young, James Harvey. "Botulism and the ripe olive scare of 1919-1920." *Bulletin of the History of Medicine* 50.3 (1976): 372-391.

Stricker, Frederick D., and Jacob Casson Geiger. "Outbreaks of botulism at Albany, Oregon, and Sterling, Colorado, February, 1924." *Public Health Reports* (1896-1970) (1924): 655-663.

Wilbur, Ray Lyman, and William Ophüls. "Botulism: A Report of Food-Poisoning Apparently Due to Eating of Canned String Beans, with Pathological Report of a Fatal Case." *Archives of Internal Medicine*, vol. 14, no. 4, 1914, pp. 589-604. Free PDF download on Google Scholar.

CHAPTER 1

Death in All Speeds: Quick to Lingering
THE SAN FRANCISCO, CALIFORNIA
BOARDING HOUSE OUTBREAK of 1902

On Wednesday evening, November 26, 1902, a meal of boiled beef and canned goods was served at a fashionable three-story boarding house located at 1600 McAllister Street in San Francisco, California. Of the twenty diners, some were permanent residents and others were local guests, including new proprietors and former owners of the building. The majority of the diners refused to eat what they considered an unsavory meal. Although botulinum toxin has no smell and no taste, the quality of the food was suspect for other reasons. A few even joked that the cook was trying to starve them in preparation for the Thanksgiving holiday the following day. Those who did eat would come to regret the decision. That meal would result in eight cases of botulism, many of which would initially go misdiagnosed. Five people survived the poisoning. Three others died of botulism over the course of the following three weeks.

The three fatal cases were treated separately by three different physicians. The first fatal case was assigned cerebral hemorrhage as a cause of death; that physician assured the newspaper readership that he was "positive he made no mistake about the diagnosis and the treatment."

The second fatal case was classified as pulmonary edema by the physician who was equally emphatic about his diagnosis. He was quoted by the newspaper as saying he was "positive the woman's death was not caused by eating poisoned meat."

The third fatality unfolded slowly, but then declined rapidly into a death spiral ending on the twenty-second day. That physician noted that his patient showed all the signs of food poisoning early in the illness; cause of death: ptomaines.

Eventually, the three physicians consulted together and agreed the fatal cases had enough similarities to reclassify the deaths as generalized food poisoning referred to in that era as 'ptomaine' poisoning. This new conclusion was still a misdiagnosis, albeit a mutually agreed upon one, but it came closer to the truth. Ultimately, it was the pathologist who conducted the autopsies who determined the actual cause of deaths was botulism caused by botulinum toxin in their shared meal. That pathologist would later come to be known as an expert in the field of botulism in the United States.

The Survivors

Charles D. Thurston, Mr. & Mrs. William C. Carpenter, Dr. Julius W. Hupfeld, and his wife, Ottilie Hupfeld, experienced botulism poisoning from the meal and displayed severe neurological symptoms but were fortunate enough to survive. Charles Thurston suffered dizziness and nervousness, but was reportedly able to continue to work, at least initially. By the time Charles saw his physician thirteen days after the meal, he was suffering with "general tiredness, great muscular weakness, making it difficult for him to walk, constipation, and had no desire to work." He also had dryness in the throat and nausea.

Mr. and Mrs. William C. Carpenter, the former proprietors of the boarding house, were "slightly ill" but were expected to recover, or so it was reported at the beginning of the episode. However, botulism can worsen by the hour. When the physician saw Mrs. Carpenter twelve days after the meal, the illness had confined her to bed. She had "general muscle weakness, lack of desire to get up, lack of appetite, constipation, and scratching and dryness in the throat."

Dr. Julius W. Hupfeld, aged sixty-four, and his twenty-two-year-old bride, Ottilie, experienced neurological symptoms similar to those of the others. About ten days after the meal, Dr. Hupfeld's symptoms were "tiredness, dizziness, lack of appetite, pronounced weakness in the legs, inability to walk two blocks, heaviness of the arms, and dryness of the mouth." Ottilie's muscles in her throat were slightly paralyzed, her eyelids were drooping from weakened muscles (ptosis), and she was constipated. Interestingly, the Hupfelds recovered adequately enough to sail to Panama on a steamship eighteen days after the food poisoning episode. Dr. Hupfeld had been widowed the year prior after a forty-year marriage. He and his young bride survived botulism and survived the Panama journey. Ottilie lived to be eighty-seven years old.

The survivors displayed the classic symptoms of botulism: dry throat, nausea, general weakness, extreme fatigue, difficulty walking, and a stubborn constipation from paralysis of the bowels. The neurological symptoms indicated that these were not cases of routine food poisonings; they were undiagnosed botulism. After all, in 1902, botulism was seldom recognized by physicians in the U.S.

The Fatalities

The three people who died after ingesting the poisonous meal included a local businessman, the bride of the new proprietor, and a male resident of the boarding house. The physical feature they all shared was having a small body with a slim build. (Many decades later researchers would correlate spread of toxin with lower muscle mass.)

The first fatality was Seth Clisby, a local businessman. The year prior, he had inherited his late father's estate, including the Eureka Warehouse near the piers at Montgomery Street and Chestnut Street. Seth was a native of Oakland and the beloved husband of Ethel Corinne (Becht) Clisby. Seth and Ethel lived in a home in the Cole Valley neighborhood about a thirty-minute walk from the boarding house on McAllister Street and Divisadero Street. On the Wednesday before Thanksgiving, Seth made a fateful decision to dine at the boarding house located between the warehouse and their home. Thanksgiving of 1902 was their third wedding anniversary.

Seth went to work on Thanksgiving Day, but when he arrived home that Thursday afternoon, he was so weak "he had to drag himself up the stairs." When he arose on Friday morning, the muscles in his face had "stiffened." Seth sought medical attention from Dr. E.J. McConnell on Friday afternoon to "find out what was the matter with him." Dr. McConnell was preparing to leave town, so he referred his patient to Dr. Donald R. Smith for follow-up over the weekend. Seth initially refused to leave Dr. McConnell's office, feeling he was desperately in need of medical attention. Dr. McConnell later told the newspapers that he telephoned Ethel about Seth's refusal to leave "and instructed her to get him home at once."

By Friday night at 10:00 PM, when her husband's symptoms had worsened, Ethel telephoned the second physician, Dr. Smith. Seth's paralysis had spread to his throat and tongue; he could not swallow and he "spoke with great difficulty." His temperature was subnormal. Dr.

Smith reported that Seth told him that "he knew he was going to die" and that he had made out a legal will.

Seth William Clisby, age twenty-nine, died on Sunday, November 30, 1902, just four days after eating the meal tainted with botulinum toxin. Seth's cause of death was initially misdiagnosed by Dr. Smith as cerebral hemorrhage; there was no suspicion of poisoning.

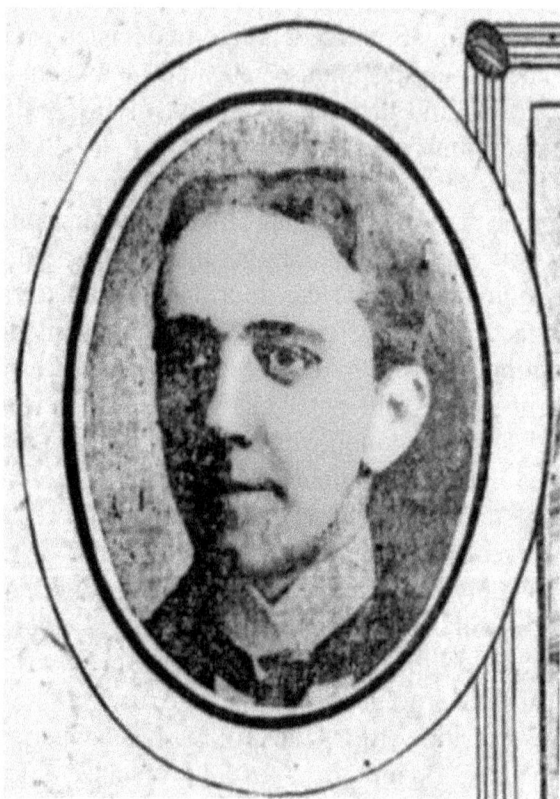

Seth William Clisby

The second fatality was Pearl Eva Cass, age twenty-one. She was the new bride of John Lewis Cass, who had purchased the boarding house on November 20, 1902, just six days before the tragedy. Eva had graduated as a stenographer from a business school in San Jose in 1898. Eva and John both worked for *The Examiner* newspaper in Marysville and had been married about six months before they moved to San Francisco.

About two days after the Wednesday meal, Eva was "compelled to take to her own bed." John told the *San Francisco Chronicle* newspaper that his wife "saw double, suffered dizziness, and also complained that her throat was sore and swollen." The newspaper reported Eva had "telephoned for her mother, who came to the house the next day, remaining long enough to convince herself that her daughter was not seriously ill."

As is often the case, those around people who are in the early stages of botulism don't consider the illness to be serious from their outside perspectives. The families of the victims of botulinum toxin poisoning often interpret the victim's descriptions of their illness as complaining when in reality, the victim is battling the most poisonous poison known to man–botulinum toxin.

Three or four days after Eva ingested the toxin, John thought "an outing would do Eva good." He took her to the Cliff House beach on the Pacific Ocean, a landmark destination less than five miles west of their boarding house.

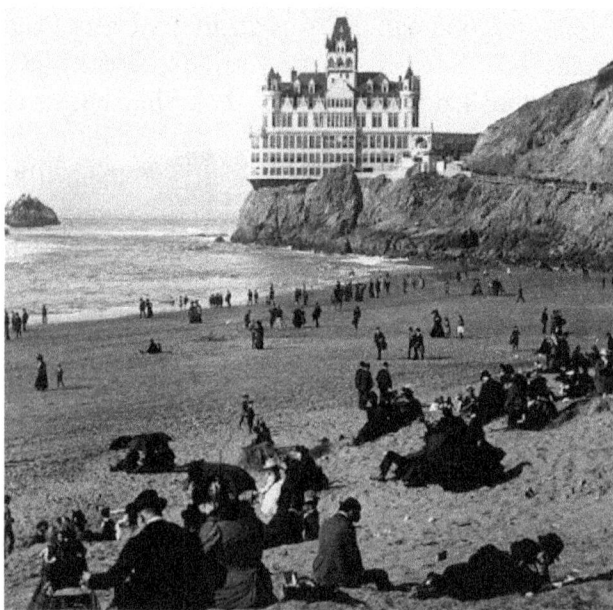

The Beach and Cliff House - San Francisco, CA - 1902

Walking long distances on a large sandy beach would have been difficult–if not impossible–for someone in the tightening grip of botulism. By this stage of the illness, Eva would have been experiencing increasingly severe muscle fatigue and generalized weakness. Likely, the physical exertion accelerated the circulation of the botulinum toxin molecules through the bloodstream and hastened the uptake of the toxin into the nerve endings, leading to more paralysis.

John recalled that his wife "suffered more or less" that first week of December, an odd description by a husband not fully appreciating the seriousness of his wife's health status. Operating a boarding house was no doubt a physically demanding job in 1902 even with help from the staff. With people renting rooms and a kitchen

8

operation feeding those boarders as well as other local diners, the work was never ending. The day before she died, Eva "complained" to her husband "of feeling general weakness" and told him that "her strength had left her during the night and that she was unable to even raise her arms." Pearl Eva Cass, age twenty-one, died on Monday, December 8, 1902 after a grueling twelve days of poisoning from botulinum toxin. The cause of death was initially misdiagnosed by her physician as "mitral insufficiency, pulmonary edema, and hysterical pneumonia."

Everett Farnum Goodyear was the third and final fatality. His death was drawn out and painful; the newspaper reported he had "lingered in the throes of pain" for almost three weeks. Everett had been a resident of the boarding house for several years. Born in Boone County, Iowa, Everett worked for the Macmillan Publishing Company in San Francisco.

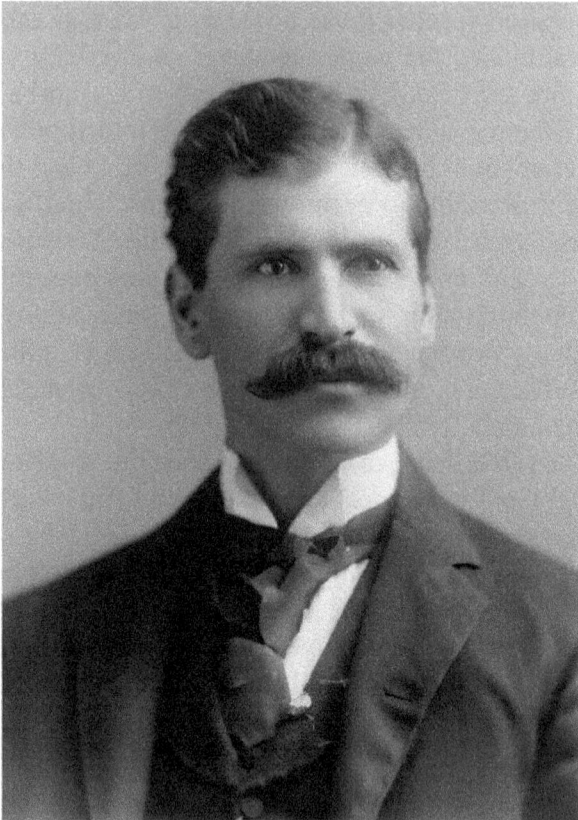

Everett Farnum Goodyear

On the seventh day after the suspect meal, Everett was quite ill, and on the ninth day, he sought medical attention at the Homeopathic Sanatorium. On the fourteenth day, Dr. Emil Otto Jellinek was called to treat Everett and found him in "great distress." Dr. Jellinek summarized the health history:

> "The patient became sick with
> symptoms of pronounced prostrations,

lack of appetite, dryness and
scratching in the throat. He could
open his eyes only with great
difficulty. He was constipated, no
urinary disturbances, no headache. On
the following day difficulty in
swallowing was present, which
increased to actually an inability to
swallow, accompanied by increasing
dryness of the mouth and pharynx and
great thirst. The voice became
hoarse, breathing and pulse
quickened. No food had been taken for
five days."

The medical literature on botulism in the United
States was exceedingly sparse at the turn of the
twentieth century. The few case reports on food
poisoning that were published in medical journals
often included abundant details, so other physicians
could learn from previous cases. In this spirit of
diligent observation, Dr. Jellinek studied his
patient's illness and described the symptoms in
great detail:

"The patient rested in a passive,
half-sitting position in bed; the
head dropped over his right shoulder.
The skin was pale and dry, expression
of the face was crestfallen. The eyes
were closed and the eyelids could be
raised with great effort about one
cm. Eye movements were free, no
diplopia, no disturbance of the
facial or trigeminus nerves. The
tongue could be voluntarily stretched
out and moved in all directions,
still the movements were retarded."

Dr. Jellinek also reported the absence of symptoms

in an effort to provide a complete clinical picture:

> "The patient could whistle, there was
> no atrophy of the tongue or lips. The
> uvula was raised only slowly, the
> pharyngeal reflexes sluggish. Speech
> was low and hoarse, and distinctly
> nasal, often unintelligible. The
> principal complaints of the patient
> were the severe dryness of the throat
> and the inability to swallow.
> Temperature 102, pulse 120-140.
> Breathing shallow – 36 per minute.
> Sensorium undisturbed."

The following day Everett worsened. Dr. Jellinek's report listed severe insomnia:

> "The prostration was even more
> pronounced and the patient not having
> slept although one-fourth of a grain
> of morphine had been administered. In
> fact, since the beginning of this
> illness the patient had slept
> scarcely two hours."

Dr. Jellinek decided to move Everett to the German Hospital where he worked as a visiting physician and could provide closer observation. He described Everett's case as "pitiful." Everett could "not swallow ice water or anything else," nor articulate distinctly. His eyelids were drooping so severely that he appeared to have his eyes shut. Dr. Jellinek had intended to "bleed the patient and inject saline solution into the blood to wash it," but Everett's pulse was too weak. He had not slept for seven days. Dr. Jellinek gave Everett an injection of morphine, and he seemed "brighter."

On the twenty-first day of the illness, Dr. Jellinek visited Everett at 10:00 PM Friday and thought he "appeared a little better." However, a few hours later, at 4:00 AM Saturday morning, Everett Farnum Goodyear, age thirty-four, "died suddenly of paralysis of the heart center." This occurred twenty-two days after ingesting botulinum toxin.

Much practical knowledge was gleaned from this 1902 botulism outbreak. First, this outbreak showed that misdiagnosis was a common error even among competent physicians. Second, the eight cases reflected a wide variation in symptoms. Third, atypical symptoms were documented such as presence of a fever and subnormal temperatures. Fourth, the randomness of recovery and fatality was astonishingly difficult to predict.

Finally, this outbreak showed how unpredictable the time course of botulism is; death could occur within days or over weeks. Seth died after four days. Eva died after twelve days. Everett died after twenty-two days.

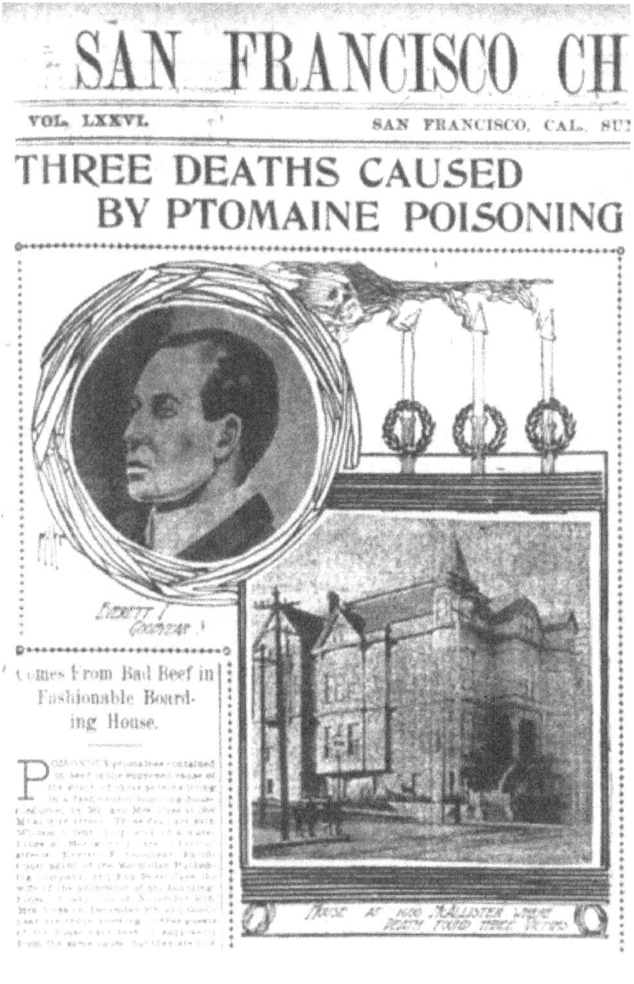
SAN FRANCISCO CH

VOL. LXXVI. SAN FRANCISCO, CAL. SU

THREE DEATHS CAUSED BY PTOMAINE POISONING

Comes From Bad Beef in Fashionable Boarding House.

Dr. Emil Otto Jellinek published an article in a medical journal the following year–*On Ptomaine Poisoning*. This is an odd title because at the end of the article the conclusion was that these ptomaine fatalities were actually botulism cases. However, in the early 1900s, doctors who researched the topic would recognize the word 'ptomaine' more readily than the word 'botulism'. The article included the pathology findings from Dr. William Ophuls, who was trained in bacteriology in Germany and employed at Stanford University as a professor of Pathology. Due to his training in Germany, where botulism had been recognized and researched since 1820, and many publications on botulism were readily available, Dr. Ophuls had the medical background and skills to recognize the fatal food poisoning cases as botulism.

The 1903 article *On Ptomaine Poisoning* is the earliest known example, in English, of an autopsy on a botulism victim performed by a physician versed in the pathology of botulism.

Dr. Ophuls would become instrumental in translating the German publications about botulism into English. Dr. E.C. Dickson, also at Stanford University, used the insights from these translated works as the foundation for his own 1918 monograph on botulism outbreaks in the United States. Dr. E.C. Dickson's book was the first book published in English about botulism. Georgina Burke worked alongside Dr. Dickson in the Laboratory of Bacteriology and Experimental Pathology Stanford University.

In his lifetime, Dr. Ophuls completed three thousand autopsies and published his statistical observations in his own book in 1926. Though Dr. Ophuls passed away in 1933, his contributions endure.

Career Ends

DEATH TAKES DOCTOR OPHULS OF STANFORD

Famous Pathologist and Dean of Medical School Succumbs; Civic Activities Are Recalled

Dr. William Ophuls, dean of the Stanford Medical School and one of the best known medical men in the State, died at the Stanford Hospital yesterday after a protracted illness.

Born sixty-two years ago in Brooklyn, N. Y., Dr. Ophuls had come to be one of the foremost pathologists in the country. His pathological research here, subsidized by the Rockefeller Institute, had been the subject of innumerable medical tracts, and formed the major part of a book that he completed shortly before his death.

STUDIED AT WURZBURG.

Dr. Ophuls studied at the University of Wurzburg in Germany, later took his master's degree at the University of Gottingen. At the latter, he was assistant professor in pathology and bacteriology for two years. He came as full profes-

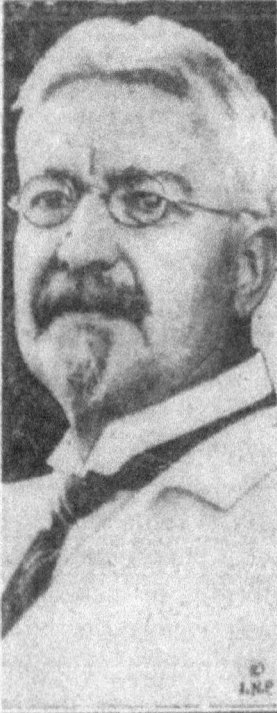

DR. WILLIAM O. HULS, dean of Stanford medical school, who died yesterday.

Dr. William Ophuls

TAKEAWAYS from
THE SAN FRANCISCO OUTBREAK

Botulism presents a distinct set of neurological symptoms that can easily be misdiagnosed when physicians lack direct experience with botulism.

Individual cases of botulism are routinely misdiagnosed.

Botulism symptoms unfold at a different pace for each patient and can present with different severities. Even when all cases are fatalities, the progression varies greatly.

Within a single botulism outbreak, patients can share common symptoms, but can also present with a different combination of symptoms among them.

Botulism symptoms wax and wane, giving hope for recovery, only to suddenly result in a fatal outcome.

Death can occur weeks after poisoning. The lower the dose, the longer the time to death, numerous animal models testing for toxicity confirm this progression.

Complete respiratory collapse from botulism can occur with little to no warning, resulting in death within minutes.

RECOGNIZING BOTULISM

CHAPTER 2

Insidious Deaths in Four Days
CUCAMONGA CANYON, CALIFORNIA
OUTBREAK of 1907

In the final days of 1906, the Carter and Abbott families gathered in Ontario, California, to celebrate the holidays and plan the wedding of their children, Mabel Carter and Charles Abbott. The gathering, which held so much promise for the families, would result in three deaths from rapidly progressing cases of botulism.

The Carters held this gathering in their home in the Ontario Colony Lands, a place lush with established orange groves about forty miles southeast of Los Angeles, California. Within a decade of construction, Ontario Colony Lands was heralded as a model of planned communities because it integrated urban and rural development. At the centerpiece was Euclid Avenue, eight miles long and two hundred feet wide with grass and pepper trees in median. By 1906, Ontario was home to about four thousand people.

Charles Abbott, Mabel Carter, and her father, Henry Carter, would share a meal together on a hike in the San Gabriel mountains and later die from an exceptionally lethal type of food poisoning within a week. Their deaths came with rapid symptom onset and little warning. Charles and Mabel's mothers, who had been joyously planning a wedding ceremony for their children, suddenly found themselves making funeral arrangements instead.

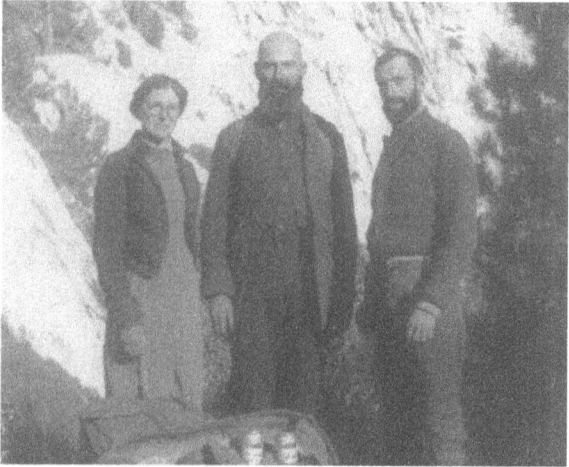

Mabel, Henry, and Charles
Image generated using MidJourney AI

As a young man, Charles Abbott worked at a grocery store in Los Angeles owned by Henry Carter, Mabel's father, and had impressed both Henry and Alvaretta, Mabel's mother. Charles would go on to meet their daughter, Mabel, and win her heart as well. By the age of twenty-three, he had moved to Artesia and held a respectable job as an engineer and machinist at the Los Alamitos sugar factory. Charles was also involved with two civic lodges: the Woodmen and the Maccabees.

Mabel, twenty-seven at the time of her engagement, was blessed with beauty and talent. She worked as a music teacher, served as a singer in the Christ Church choir, and was prominent in the musical circles of Los Angeles.

The Carters hosted Charles, his brother Albert, and their mother, Mrs. Abbott, over the holiday break. This was a chance for the families to get to know one another better. During the previous two years, Henry Carter had become a prominent orange grove rancher in Ontario, California. It was a prosperous time; orange growers had adapted a variety of navel oranges from Washington State to Southern California, and the industry was burgeoning from the introduction of the railroad.

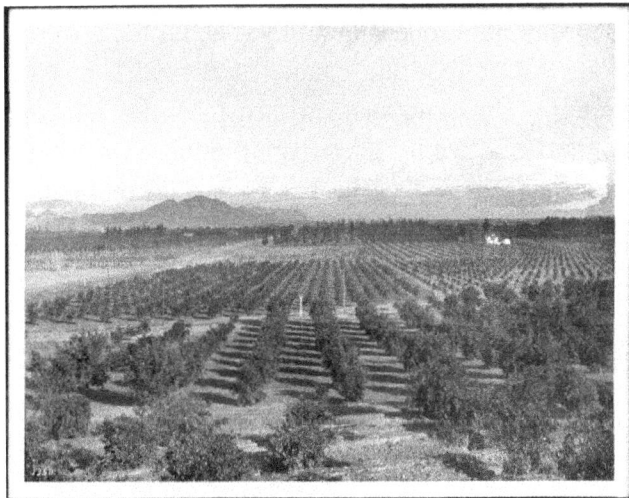

Group of citrus groves in southern California, ca.1900

During the 1906 holiday visit, Charles mentioned that he had never been in the snow. Even at sixty-three years old, Henry was a mountain climbing enthusiast. He proposed, practically insisted, that he take Charles and Mabel on a hiking trip through Cucamonga Canyon to the nearby peaks of the San Gabriel mountains, so Charles could experience snow or "the Beautiful," as the snow was referred to colloquially. Henry and Mabel decided that, not only should Charles wade in the fresh snow, but he should also experience a real snowball fight.

Cucamonga Canyon was roughly an eight-mile trip by horse-drawn buggy from Ontario. The three adventurers, Henry, Mabel, and Charles, packed provisions of fresh food, leftover home-cooked meals, a can of condensed milk, and two cans of pork and beans.

They set off for a few days of hiking up the mountain to see the snowline. After their arrival on Saturday, they hiked in and pitched a tent. Weary from travel, they ate canned pork and beans for dinner. Unbeknownst to them, their dinner contained a deadly toxin. Botulinum toxin has no smell and no taste. The hikers had no inclination that trouble was ahead for them.

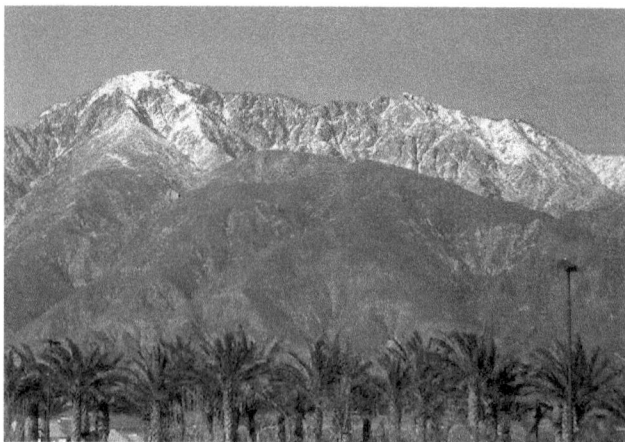

Cucamonga Peak

A winter storm moved in, forcing the trio to break camp and take shelter in a nearby cabin they found unoccupied. The same day they experienced the onset of symptoms from the toxin in the previous night's dinner. Henry was the first to feel ill. Feeling as though he was suffering from one of his usual "bilious attacks"—an issue common for him—he remained at the camp while Mabel and Charles went mountain climbing. Henry also complained of double vision.

Charles also experienced vision issues. Though he was a seasoned marksman, during shooting practice he was unable to hit his mark. Later, when he tried to split firewood, he could not reliably strike the stick. No one went mountain climbing on that day. The men made a joke of their double vision and attributed their eyesight issues to not being accustomed to the higher altitude of the mountain. As an experienced hiker, Henry likely knew that a high altitude could cause vision issues.

By Tuesday, New Year's Day, Henry was quite ill. Mabel and Charles wanted to return home that morning. Henry insisted that the couple "tramp up the canyon as had been arranged." Mabel and Charles left early, shortly after breakfast, and had a delightful climb to the snowline without any unusual physical effort.

The *San Bernardino County Sun* newspaper reported, "They got an early start, and when far up the mountain lost their way, and it was not until the shadows commenced to settle over the canyon, and the weather turned to freezing, that they finally managed to get their bearings." Mabel and Charles made it back to camp after 3:00 PM and told Henry that they had "the times of their lives." They made the climb successfully, even enjoyably, despite the mild neurological symptoms that they were already experiencing.

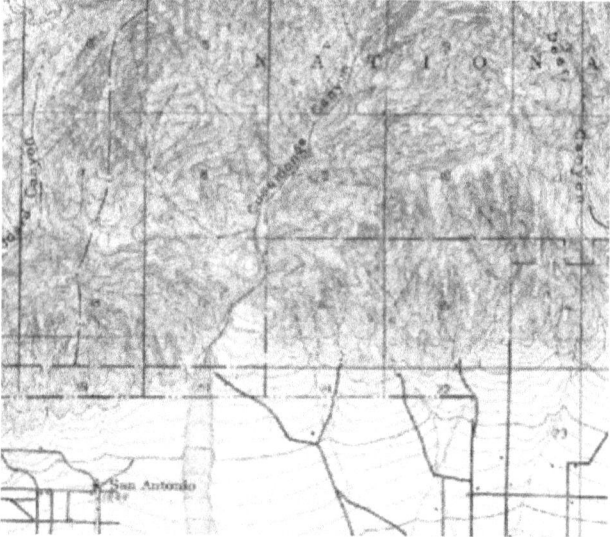

Cucamonga Canyon Map 1910

After their hike, Mabel and Charles ate the second can of pork and beans. Henry was already too ill to eat, and in need of immediate medical attention. Mabel and Charles managed to get the horse hitched to their buggy. The group arrived home at 6:00 PM Tuesday night. Henry could no longer walk upon arrival and had to be carried from the buggy to the house. Mabel and Charles were fatigued, but still mobile.

Dr. Christopher Sheppard, the family physician, was summoned to the house and arrived inside of the hour. He immediately ascertained how critical the situation was for Henry and called upon other physicians to join him. Henry was the only one in the party who appeared visibly ill, although Mabel and Charles reported slight vision disturbances and a sense of fatigue. The couple attributed their fatigue to their mountain exercise. After dining on a hearty meal Tuesday night, Mabel told her mother, "I am simply all in and must get to bed. Let's not do the dishes tonight. Leave them until tomorrow morning and I will do them myself."

Early Wednesday morning, around 4:00 AM, Mabel was "alarmingly ill." She told her mother then that she was dying. Charles was called to assist in caring for her.

People who experience acute poisoning from botulinum toxin often express deep convictions that reflect they know, without a doubt, they are actively in the process of dying. Because the rapid onset of botulism is unexpected, those tending to the victim often can't conceive that death is imminent. Caregivers realize the patient is ill, but often don't grasp the gravity of the situation.

The doctors and family did everything medically possible to save the lives of Mabel, Charles, and Henry. The *San Bernardino County Sun* newspaper described how Mabel's suffering:

> "Hour after hour the physicians worked over the stricken girl and men, never for a moment stopping to rest until nature could not stand the strain [any] longer, and other physicians were called. Friends also assisted, following the instructions of the doctors, faithfully, but gradually the symptoms of poisoning developed . . . ."

The patients' stomachs were emptied and cleansed by lavage. An attempt at purging was a failure. Hypodermoclysis (administering fluids subcutaneously instead of through an IV) was attempted to dilute the poison in the blood and help with urine excretion. Strychnia, tropia, digitalis, caffeine, and camphor were used. Coffee and whiskey were administered in the rectum to flush out poisons held in the colon. These were standard procedures for flushing the body of poisons.

Mabel, Charles, and Henry developed similar symptoms over a short span of time. The gastrointestinal symptoms usually associated with food poisoning were entirely absent. None of them had sensory disturbances or fevers. The first complaint for all three was a disturbance of vision; they reported a "mistiness while looking in certain directions." Henry and Mabel had ptosis: their upper eyelids were drooping. Once circulating in the bloodstream, botulinum toxin commonly damages the oculomotor nerve, which results in weakening the levator palpebrae superioris muscles responsible for raising and lowering the eyelids.

Charles did not display ptosis initially. He did develop a thickness in his speech and difficulty swallowing. A swollen tongue is a common symptom of botulism. He tried to communicate by writing, but his penmanship was illegible due to flaccid paralysis of his fingers and hands. Botulinum toxin also damages the nerves that control the muscles used in speaking and swallowing. It would soon become impossible for any of them to swallow. Dr. Sheppard attempts to capture a teachable moment as he described their other symptoms:

> "Difficulty breathing was also a
> constant and common symptom, and a
> general fatigue of muscular power,
> the whole picture being one of a
> gradually developing motor paralysis.
> A profuse secretion of mucus in the
> throat was a source of great
> distress, as owing to the paralyzed
> condition of the throat muscles it
> was impossible to get rid of it."

Botulinum toxin also damages the nerves that signal the diaphragm muscles necessary for breathing. The general fatigue results in flaccid paralysis; it occurs when nerves all over the body are damaged and unable to signal the muscles to contract.

Near the end, the pulse of each patient was "little altered except for a marked quickening" that happened upon any movement of the body. The body temperatures were normal or subnormal. The intestines were paralyzed from nerve damage, thus preventing attempts at purgation. Dr. Sheppard described the mental condition of the patients as "clear and undisturbed" except for an "unnatural irritability" when they made an effort to speak and could not be understood. Henry also attempted to communicate through writing, but his handwriting was illegible. The flaccid paralysis associated with botulism became so severe that even the minimal effort of holding a pencil became impossible for Henry.

Mabel Carter died suddenly while resting in her mother's arms around 4:00 AM on Thursday morning. She passed away quietly; the "exact moment or manner of death not being observed."

Death occurred just twenty-four hours after Mabel was considered alarmingly ill.

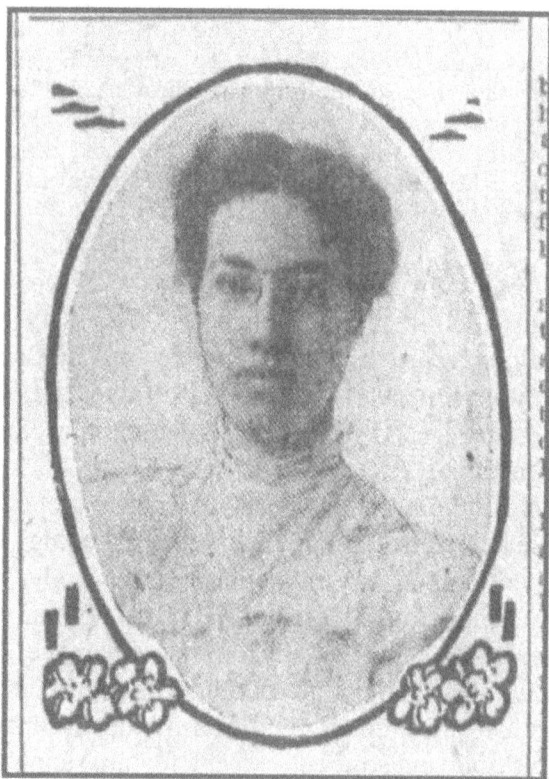

Mabel Carter

At the time of Mabel's death early Thursday, the doctors felt the situation was not hopeless for Henry and Charles. However, later in the day, their "conditions changed rapidly for the worse." The news was "broken gently to Mrs. Carter, who though advanced in years, bravely faced the situation." At fifty-seven years old, Alvaretta Carter faced both the grief of losing her only child and the prospect of becoming a widow. Still, she tended to Charles and Henry throughout their continued declines.

By noon Thursday, Charles became severely ill. He stayed upright and mobile as long as possible, telling the others that if he ever laid down, he would never get up. However, at 4:00 PM, his condition forced him to the bed. The botulinum toxin had, by then, spread throughout his body, making it impossible for him to support his own weight regardless of any power of will. Once botulinum toxin has spread systemically through the body, willpower alone will not suffice. It becomes physically impossible for flaccid muscles to support a body.

Charles Abbott died Friday morning around 10:30 AM. His mother and brother were still at the Carter's home. His father had traveled by train in a futile attempt to make it to his Charles's deathbed before he passed. The physician's report on Charles explained that "he seemed to be in a safe condition, pulse and respiration being good when breathing suddenly failed and he was dead in a few minutes." Neither the bedfast patient nor the physician recognized the imminent danger presented by the poison.

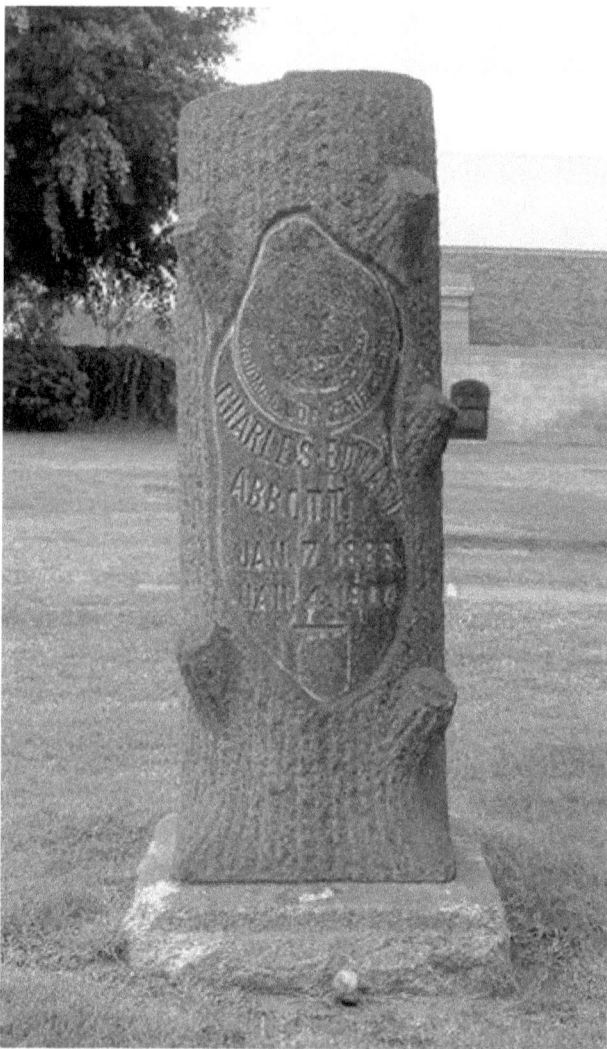

Grave marker for Charles Edward Abbott

Henry lingered until Friday afternoon, his wife at his bedside. He was unable to speak or write. Prior to his demise, his condition improved slightly. With some difficulty, he was able to swallow; whereas earlier, swallowing had been impossible.

His case again illustrates that botulism symptoms can wax and wane, causing momentary hope the condition is improving when in fact, death is imminent. Henry Sylvester Carter died of botulism on Friday, January 4, 1907; the death was attributed to "general exhaustion."

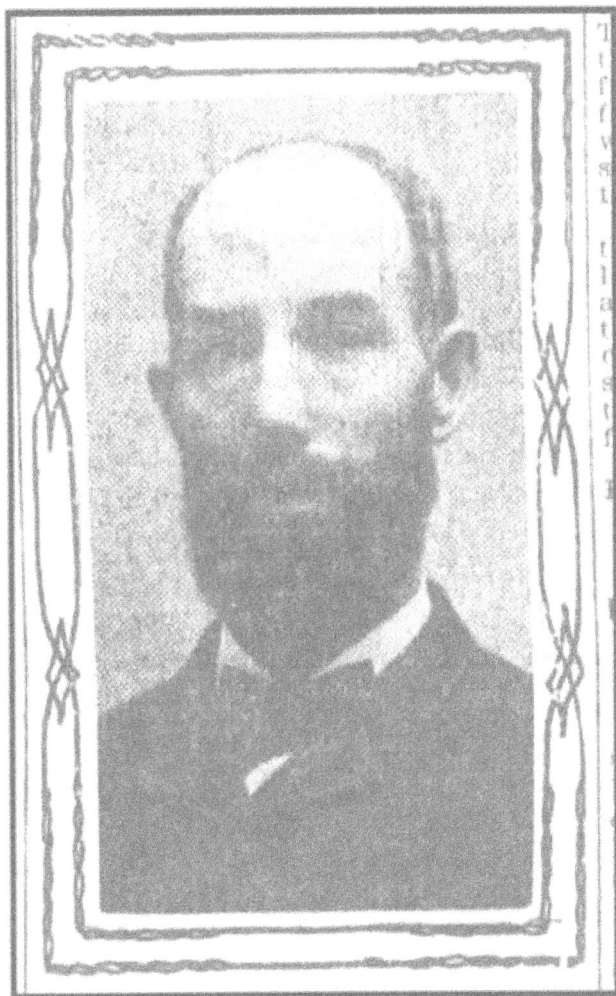

Henry Sylvester Carter

Alvaretta Van Pelt Carter began the new year in 1907 as a widow who had lost both her husband and her only child to a tragic disease. She grieved alongside Charles's mother, both of them having lost dearly. The newspaper commented on the unfortunate situation, noting "singularly pathetic is the attachment of the two bereaved mothers, both in their grief trying to console each other."

Dr. Sheppard published his observations in a medical journal to advance the understanding of this strange type of food poisoning. He explained that "these cases were exceptional in their insidious development." He was perplexed that there was an "entire absence of the gasto- intestinal symptoms" usually seen at the outset of food poisoning. To the best of his knowledge, a diagnosing physician would look for the first definite symptoms of food poisoning including "chills, giddiness, faintness, headache, or pain in some part of the body" followed soon by abdominal pain, vomiting, and purging. Dr. Sheppard remarked:

> "Other symptoms, chiefly referred to the nervous system, may follow but are irregular, such as tingling, numbness, convulsive moments, cramps, etc. Some such symptoms have been observed in a number of cases; others only in solitary instances, as that from what I find in the scanty literature on the subject within my reach. The cases we had to deal with were of an unusual character."

Due to the limited knowledge of botulism in the United States in 1907, Dr. Sheppard would not have realized that botulism cases were notorious for being of "an usual character" because of the large variation in symptoms that present, even within the same outbreak.

Later, the unopened cans of pork and beans from the hike were inspected and "in appearance, taste and smell pronounced to be very good." The remains of the actual pork and beans eaten by the hikers were left behind at the cabin, which happened to be owned by John Bunnell, a typesetter at the local newspaper. John learned about the tragedy while preparing the story about the deaths of the hikers for publication. As he typeset each line of the story, John wondered where exactly the ill-fated hikers had sought shelter from the storm. He knew there were only two cabins in Cucamonga Canyon: his cabin and Hugo Sontag's cabin.

John went to the mountains himself the next week and was shocked to discover that the ill-fated trio of hikers had overnighted in his cabin. He then visited with his only neighbor, Hugo, to share his discovery. Hugo shared his own tragic story; eight of his best hens had mysteriously died the same week the hikers died.

John Bunnell pieced the two fatal events together. In the chicken coop, John and Hugo found an empty can of pork and beans that fatally poisoned the hiking party and Hugo's chickens. Botulinum toxin type A causes a condition in chickens called limberneck. The damaged nerves cause flaccid paralysis of the muscles, especially the neck muscles. Hugo's chickens were physically unable to hold up their heads, and they died from paralysis of the diaphragm, just as people experience. The chickens suffocated to death from a lack of oxygen.

Reflecting on the earlier events at the Carter home, the newspaper recounted the physicians' puzzlement:

> "The case has different features than any they have yet dealt with. All three of the unfortunate party were attacked with a double vision, a numbness of the limbs and a paralysis of the tongue. A few hours before death the eyelids closed and it was impossible for them to open them. None of the three experienced any pain and the case throughout is most puzzling."

The deaths were classified as "ptomaine poisoning." An autopsy was performed on Charles Abbott. In a 1907 publication by Dr. Stanley Black, a professor of pathology at the College of Medicine of the University of Southern California, he stated the following:

> "The pathologic lesions . . . are usually ecchymoses in the gastrointestinal mucosa, and also in the pleura pericardium and peritoneum. Fluid blood is often found in the heart cavities and congestion and cloudy swelling of the parenchymal organs [kidneys, adrenal glands, liver, spleen, and pancreas]. Besides these lesions, there are sometimes found certain degenerative changes in the nerve cells of the brain and spinal cord."

In 1907, ptomaine poisoning was a blanket term used to describe any general food poisoning. It would be eleven years before a medical textbook on botulism would be published in English. While the U.S. medical journals in the early 1900s used the term "ptomaine poisoning" almost exclusively, over time the terms 'botulism' and "ptomaine poisoning" were used interchangeably. Gradually, the term "ptomaine" was dropped from use.

Gradually, the medical community recognized that specific neurological symptoms were associated with botulism. Within a few years, the deaths in the Cucamonga Canyon outbreak were reevaluated and determined to be the result of botulism based on the neurological symptoms and the lethality of the toxin to chickens. Dr. Sheppard's medical publication, even with his inaccurate diagnosis, was a key publication helping the medical community develop a clearer understanding of botulism. This was not to be the last time that chickens with limberneck disease (aka avian botulism) aided in a botulism diagnosis.

Interestingly, in the Cucamonga Canyon botulism outbreak, the first person to become ill, the older man, was the last person to die. The younger man was considered ill, but not in imminent danger, then died within minutes. His entire symptomatic illness lasted about eighteen hours; he did not take the mild symptoms of botulism seriously during the previous four days. The young woman died exactly one day after her severe symptoms manifested; and, she intuitively knew she was dying. Everyone in the party died within five days of their consumption of botulinum toxin, two of the fatal cases had mild enough symptoms that they were able to hike even after initial onset of issues.

There is simply no frame of reference for individuals who develop botulism poisoning. The intensity of the poison is incomprehensible as the bloodstream carries the toxin to every organ and every nerve in the human body. No other substance in the world comes remotely close to the lethality of botulinum toxin. Few, if any, botulism victims know what to expect from the disease; it is incomparable to any other illness experienced by human beings. Perhaps this is why so many victims have such a strong sense of their impending deaths? Ironically, others seem to approach their fatal outcomes with denial or stoicism, suspended in disbelief that an invisible killer could strike without warning.

Dr. Sheppard described the swift and stealthy nature of this outbreak as "insidious." Botulism is most definitely insidious, and most definitely deadly.

TAKEAWAYS from
THE CUCAMONGA CANYON
OUTBREAK

Botulism symptoms unfold at a different pace for each patient and can also present with different severities for each patient. Even when all cases are fatal outcomes, the progression varies greatly.

Within a single botulism outbreak, patients can share some symptoms in common, but can also present with a different combination from one another.

Botulism patients often underestimate their condition's severity; sudden decline and death can surprise both patient and physician.

Complete respiratory collapse from botulism can happen with little to no warning, resulting in death within minutes.

Toward the end, botulism patients often verbalize that they feel as if they are dying even though the observable symptoms do not indicate the impending fatal outcome.

The chickens that were fed the food tainted with botulinum toxin died of botulism.

CHAPTER 3

Ruby is Recovering, Ruby is Gone
THE STANFORD SORORITY
OUTBREAK of 1913

Just before the holiday season of 1913 began in earnest, the young women of Pi Beta Phi women's fraternity house at Stanford University hosted a special farewell dinner to celebrate the end of their fall semester. Contaminated green beans in one dish prepared for the celebration would lead to twelve of the celebrants falling ill of which eight were hospitalized. One of the eight died. Yet the outbreak and subsequent heartbreaking death of Ruby Lynch served as a catalyst for botulinum toxin research in the early twentieth century.

On November 25, 1913, after a trip to the mountains to gather decorative holly, the young women of Pi Beta Phi pitched in to prepare their celebratory meal. It was a Sunday, their cook's regular day off, so the young women worked together, fixing a meal of cold dishes. One of the women contributed home-canned green beans, which were used as the main ingredient in a cold wax bean salad and were later determined to be the source of the botulinum toxin. Twenty-four young women ate the dish, and twelve fell ill. (A male student waiter and Mrs. Benson, the house mother, were also reported to be slightly ill, but were not hospitalized.)

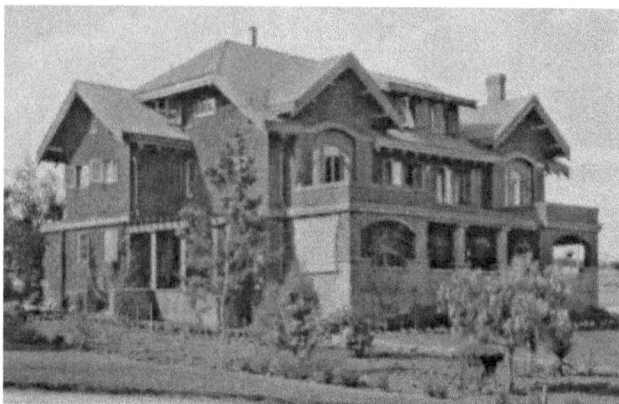

Pi Beta Phi house, Leland Stanford Jr. University, 1913

Ruby Lynch, age twenty-two, was pursuing her Master's degree in Mathematics at the time of the tragedy. When Leland Stanford Jr. University opened in 1891 and offered free tuition, it was one of the few universities in the country that allowed women to pursue advanced degrees. Jane Stanford insisted that the university she helped establish to honor the untimely death of her young son would be co-educational from the start. She also capped the female enrollment at five hundred. In 1913, Ruby Lynch was one of those five hundred women.

At first, the illness afflicting the eight young women hospitalized puzzled the scientists and physicians at Stanford. While the women had symptoms in common with each other, there was also a great deal of variety in the combinations of symptoms. Dr. Ray Lyman Wilbur, Dean of Stanford University School of Medicine, oversaw the treatments. Additionally, Dr. William Ophuls, the pathology professor at Stanford, is thought to have been instrumental in confirming the diagnosis of botulism.

POISONING OF GIRLS PUZZLING SCIENTISTS

STANFORD UNIVERSITY, Dec. 10. Stanford's scientists are baffled by the strange illness, botulism, which poisoned 10 sorority girls and others and

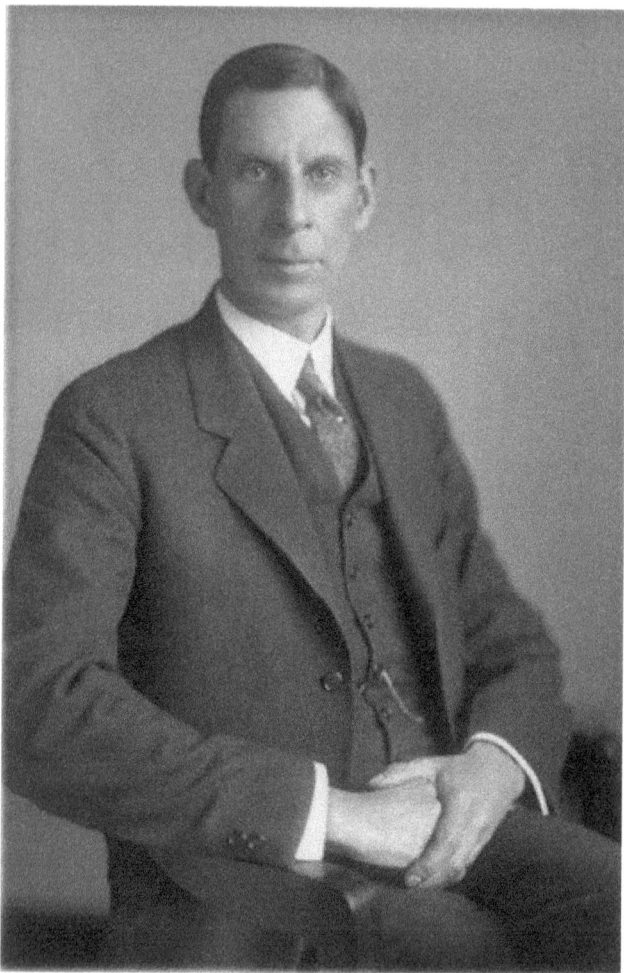

Dr. Ray Lyman Wilbur

Both doctors had experience that made them uniquely qualified to diagnose botulism, including training in Germany–a place where botulism had been recognized by the medical community since the early 1800s. In 1910, Dr. Wilbur had seen patients afflicted with botulism during his sabbatical in Cologne, Germany. In 1902, Dr.

Ophuls had diagnosed botulism after conducting autopsies on the victims of the San Francisco boarding house tragedy.

Despite the wide variety of symptoms commonly seen with botulism poisoning, and that were indeed seen in this case, Dr. Wilbur was able to make an accurate diagnosis within a week. Throughout the outbreak, Dr. Wilbur would keep accurate reporting of the progression of the illnesses within his patients, noting a wide variety and a slow manifestation of symptoms, stating, "The gradual onset of the symptoms and their marked variability are the most striking features."

Gradual onset of symptoms occurs because as botulinum toxin circulates through the bloodstream, more and more toxin molecules are taken up into the nerves. Once a nerve is damaged, it cannot signal the muscle to contract; therefore, each day, more and more new symptoms develop and initial symptoms worsen. Even the literature of 1913 documented a case where botulinum toxin was found circulating in the bloodstream one week after exposure. This circulating toxin creates a continuous and ongoing poisoning.

Dr. Wilbur also reported, "The complaint of seeing double and of the mist passing over the eyes was comparatively common." Vision disturbances are usually, but not always, the first symptom of botulism.

This unpredictable variety of symptoms documented in a botulism outbreak creates a diagnostic challenge when a single case presents. Dr. Wilbur acknowledged how difficult the diagnosis would have been if these cases had presented individually rather than as a group. He stated,

> "It is easy to see how a sporadic case could be readily overlooked or confused for various other conditions . . . The isolated case is the one that is most apt to lead to confusion and misdiagnosis."

Back then, and even now, variability of symptoms and disease progression regularly lead to misdiagnosis, especially by physicians who have never encountered botulism or diligently studied the disease.

During the course of the outbreak, the condition of the patients cycled through periods of stabilization, improvement, and worsening health. This waxing and waning as the disease progressed made it challenging for the attending physicians to grasp which patients were the most seriously ill. Dr. Wilbur reported:

> "In the patients seen by me there was a wide variation in the severity of the disease, some having only transient disturbance of vision or swallowing, others such complaints as: jaws seemed very tired, apparent inability to chew food, tongue seemed hard to move, sleepy all the time, could not walk fast, throat filled up with mucus all the time, tried to attend classes, legs and arms were almost powerless, hard work climbing stairs, throat felt as if there was a shelf in it beyond which food could not pass but it did not hurt."

Dr. Wilbur stressed that the intensity of symptoms varied from severe to mild and also the pace of disease varied as it unfolded. He shared his wisdom by warning his medical colleagues,

> "Throughout you must be constantly reminded that the symptoms may be extremely acute and followed by an early death or they may be gradually unfolded in their entirety or only one or two characteristic evidences may appear."

In other words, botulism runs the gamut from a quick death to a deceptively slow death. Additionally, there may only be one or two symptoms instead of a checklist of many symptoms.

With such a large number of people affected in this outbreak, Dr. Wilbur had the opportunity to document atypical symptoms such as non-symmetrical paralysis. Another atypical symptom that Dr. Wilbur noticed was a loss of hearing due to damage of the auditory nerves. He stated, "The girls at times, [had] difficulty hearing." Both asymmetrical paralysis and hearing loss are not generally associated with botulism and therefore can lead physicians to shifting away from a botulism diagnosis.

Dr. Wilbur made an astute observation that two opposite symptoms can occur and both are indicative of botulism. As a result of nerve damage, tear ducts may respond either with an abundance of tears or a complete loss of tears:

> "Dry mouth is accompanied apparently by a paralysis of secretory activity of many glands (parotid enlarged at times) extending in some patients even to the lacrimal glands, so that Schumacher reports the inability of a woman to shed tears when told of her husband's death. At times tears are secreted freely, and, in one of our patients, the eyes appear watery."

The disturbing sensation of suffocation is often listed as a symptom of botulism, referred to as *air hunger*. Severe botulism can cause a frightening sensation when the diaphragm muscles become paralyzed and render the victim unable to draw in the necessary breath to survive. This too was documented by Dr. Wilbur:

> "the patient complained of a dry throat and annoying thirst. There were periods of a sense of suffocation with a vague feeling of unrest and as if there might be difficulty in getting the next breath."

This paralysis of diaphragm muscles can happen quite suddenly, resulting in a swift death. However, when the paralysis advances slowly, it creates a constant and unrelenting sense of fear and panic, as if each breath might be the last.

Dr. Wilbur also described neck weakness in his patients in a way that echoed the symptoms of chickens that are poisoned by botulinum toxin and develop *limberneck*, a commonly fatal condition that weakens the neck muscles making the birds' heads go completely limp and flop to the ground.

In humans, neck weakness from botulism presents in the following manner:

> "On the twelfth day the patient was able to move her head, but unable to lift it except when she took hold of the braids for hair and pulled her head forward."

As the toxin spreads throughout the body, the disease advances and reveals an unfolding clinical picture. The slow and unpredictable demise of Miss Ruby Lynch–the sole fatality in the outbreak–progressed with a wide variety of symptoms. Dr. Wilbur wrote:

> "There was no headache or vomiting; urination and apparently as usual. On the fourth morning the patient was unable to eat because of the inability to swallow. There was no pain. Later on in the day she swallowed with difficulty. On the sixth morning her mouth was dry and there was considerable thirst, no abdominal colic, no appetite, marked asthenia [physical weakness and fatigue], with muscular power in the left arm less than normal. Voice was slightly nasal with inability to articulate distinctly. There was ptosis of both upper lids; both pupils were dilated but reactive to light, with normal fundi. The breath was foul, tongue coated and it and the pharynx covered with sticky, whitish, viscid mucus. There was considerable edema of the uvula."

While the health of a botulism patient may appear stable, the clinical condition actually waxes and wanes, creating a false sense of stability or improvement. It is commonly reported for a patient to be unable to swallow and, a few hours later, be able to eat simple food. This was the case with Ruby:

> "The condition did not change very much [in the] next few days except that the patient felt very weak, wasn't able to raise the head without help, at times could swallow well, at other times was able to take the simplest food, and the pulse became more rapid and dicrotic. Blood pressure was normal. At one time she became quite talkative and complained that her jaws did not open naturally and she could not see well but for the most part she was quiet and slightly depressed."

Ruby Lynch was two thousand miles from home. She likely had not seen her parents since school had commenced several months prior. Anyone in her vulnerable position experiencing such life-threatening symptoms would understandably be depressed and scared. Another possible cause for Ruby's depression may have been from botulinum toxin infiltrating her brain. Her only solace was that her Pi Beta Phi sisters were hospitalized with her. Dr. Wilbur described Ruby's mounting challenges,

"On the tenth day she brought up with
very much difficulty some mucus which
had been interfering greatly with her
throat and had a period in the
afternoon when she was unable to
swallow, had difficulty in breathing
and cold extremities."

Ruby's muscles became more paralyzed by the minute. Her vascular system was compromised, causing her circulation to be poor, thus the cold extremities. Her caretakers tried to provide her nourishment as she had not been able to swallow in days. Dr. Wilbur explained:

"Later on she was able to take an
eggnog, but complained of a
spontaneous choking sensation. In the
night to the distress from these
attacks was added the inability to
breathe with the nose."

Medical reports often detail how botulism patients experience attacks and even collapse from either complete flaccid paralysis or a semi-coma, only to stabilize and then die suddenly within a day. In the case of Ruby, her condition rapidly deteriorated:

"Some relief from the choking,
breathless sensation was gained by
swabbing the throat.... After a
period of chills, great restlessness,
choking sensation, increasing
temperature and higher pulse rate
together with the signs of hypostatic

pneumonia, the patient had a collapse from which she recovered on the administration by Dr. Williams of an intravenous transfusion of normal salt solution. She vomited later considerable amount of blood and although her breathing became more superficial, her weakness more evident, the sensorium remained perfectly intact."

Ruby Lynch was thought to be coming through the episode when she took a turn for the worse. At this point, Ruby began a downward spiral towards her death. In contrast, the *Ames Tribune* newspaper assured the hometown community of Ruby's condition, relaying,

"No serious results ensued and she has been heard from several times since that date and was getting along all right."

Ruby had assured her loved ones back home in Iowa that she was improving. The *Ames Evening Times* newspaper reported, "A letter written by Ruby herself on Wednesday of last week was received here in which she said that she was improving and that there was no cause for alarm." At the time Ruby wrote the letter, she was struggling to keep her eyelids open and was experiencing muscular weakness as well as breathing difficulties. Still, Ruby remained naively optimistic about her prognosis despite her fears.

Ruby Lynch died on the fifteenth day of her illness after a two-week battle with botulism. On December 9, 1913, a telegram was sent to the

Lynch family in Iowa with the message "Ruby is gone."

Sadly, her mother did not arrive in time to see her only daughter before she died in the hospital. Mrs. Lynch was enroute by train from Ames, Iowa, to Palo Alto, California–a two-thousand-mile journey. Mrs. Teresa Russell, an English teacher at Stanford University, was by Ruby's side when she died at 6:00 AM. Mrs. Russell was a longtime friend of Mrs. Lynch from their shared days living in Villisca, Iowa where Ruby was born. The Lynch family lived there for fifteen years before they moved to Ames. (In 1912, Villisca gained unfortunate notoriety when a killer bludgeoned a family of eight to death with an ax; two of the murdered children were students who Ruby had tutored in math.)

Ruby's attending physicians later stated, "There was very little difference for some time in the severity of the clinical picture between the fatal case and some of the others." The *Daily Palo Alto* newspaper reported, "The death of Miss Lynch was unexpected. Yesterday she was reported better and a telegram to that effect was sent to Denver to her mother Mrs. Dr. L.J. Lynch who is speeding west from her home in Ames, Iowa."

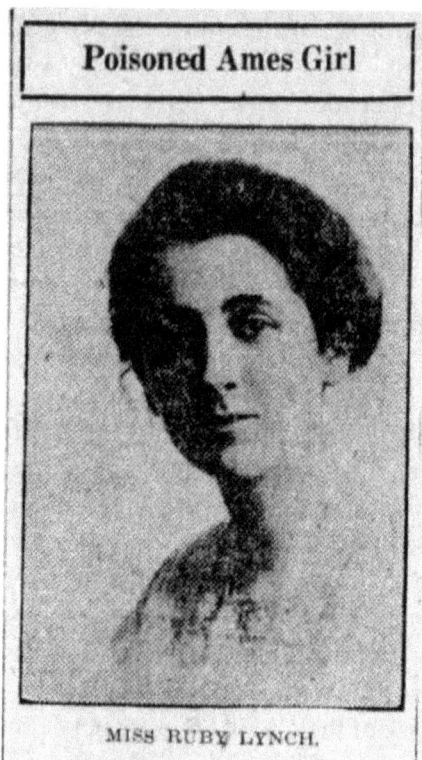

Poisoned Ames Girl

MISS RUBY LYNCH.

Ruby M. Lynch

Dr. Wilbur and Dr. Ophuls made a seminal contribution to botulism literature in 1914 when they co-authored a 15-page clinical report published in the Archives of Internal Medicine. The publication–*Botulism: A Report of Food-Poisoning Apparently due to Eating of Canned String Beans, with pathological Report of a Fatal Case*–was especially informative because the authors included the pathological report on the botulism fatality. Sharing these details with the medical community was vital to advancing the understanding of the complexity of botulism.

The length of a fatal botulism illness is difficult to predict because fatal botulism can unfold deceivingly slow then shockingly rapid. The symptoms can occur gradually over days and weeks, but then within minutes lead to death. Sudden paralysis of the diaphragm muscles–which results in immediate death–is common in severe botulism. In Ruby's case, her physicians described her rapid demise: "She died following her respiratory disturbance apparently due to sudden paralysis of the diaphragm, since the heart continued to beat for some time."

Ruby Lynch's death led to thorough documentation of a misunderstood disease, which was then published as a medical article by a reputable physician at a renowned university. This medical knowledge led to more food poisoning cases being recognized and accurately diagnosed as botulism. Had this large botulism outbreak happened in a home setting instead of a university with access to medical experts versed in botulism, this seminal contribution to science might not have occurred.

RECOGNIZING BOTULISM

TAKEAWAYS from
THE STANFORD UNIVERSITY OUTBREAK

There is variability in the symptoms even within the same botulism outbreak.

Within a single botulism outbreak, patients can share some symptoms, but can also present with different combinations.

Botulism symptoms wax and wane, giving hope for recovery, only to suddenly result in a fatal outcome.

Botulism patients often underestimate the severity of their condition; a patient can experience a sudden decline, then die to the surprise of the physician.

Severity waxes and wanes. Victims have temporary improvements before rapid declines in status, resulting in fatal outcomes.

Complete respiratory collapse from botulism can happen with little to no warning, resulting in death within minutes.

Death can occur up to two weeks (or more) after ingestion of poison.

Neither severity of symptoms nor early symptom onset are reliable predictors about

the recovery potential or the probability of
fatality of a botulism patient

CHAPTER 4

Physician Survives Botulism
THE DAWSON CITY,
YUKON TERRITORY
OUTBREAK of 1919

Who better to describe the symptoms of botulinum toxin poisoning than a physician who survived a severe case of botulism? In 1917, Dr. J.A.R. Glancy journeyed to Dawson City in the Yukon Territory–the hub of the Klondike Gold Rush of 1896. Dr. Glancy, age twenty-eight, took over the practice of Dr. Chapman, who had left to serve on the front in the Great War. Dr. Glancy was employed as the camp doctor for Yukon Gold Company mining. He had arranged to write his thesis to complete his M.D. while in Dawson City– a town once known as "The Paris of the North." Dawson City had an instant population of forty thousand at the peak of the, but by the time Dr. Glancy arrived, Dawson City had become a small mining town with a population of less than one thousand people and the small claims held by individual miners were consolidated by one large mining company, the Guggenheims of New York.

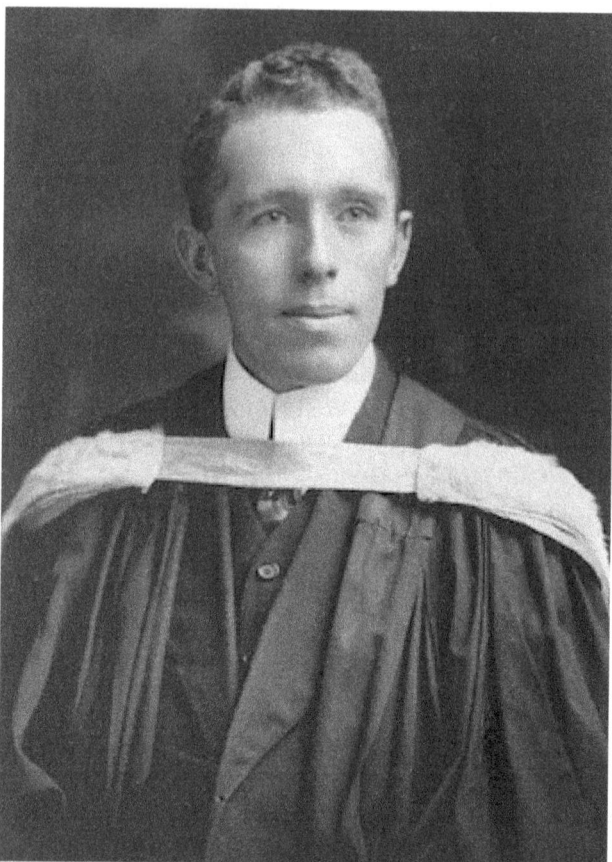

J.A.R. Glancy, MD University of Toronto 1917

Dr. Glancy had not planned to experience life-threatening botulism and discuss the disease firsthand as his thesis topic, but that was exactly his circumstance in 1919. His thesis was the first written on botulism in Canada; it made a seminal contribution to the medical field that remains unprecedented even today. Dr. Glancy recorded a plethora of details about his illness, and two dozen other men. This detailed record allowed the medical community to better understand the complexities and nuances of botulism as the illness progresses to fatality or recovery. Dr. Glancy even conducted six-month and twelve-month follow-up interviews with the men who recovered from botulism.

On Wednesday, May 22, 1919, a noon meal was served at Camp A54 at Hunker Creek outside of Dawson City. The Yukon Gold Company hosted a banquet to celebrate Victoria Day in honor of the birthday of Queen Victoria of the United Kingdom of Britain and Ireland. Victoria Day was a national holiday marked by carnivals, parades, and sporting events. Of the forty-one men who unknowingly partook of the celebratory meal tainted with botulinum toxin. Twelve men died. Twenty-three men were sickened and six felt no ill effects.

Dr. Glancy dined with the miners that fateful day and was one of the lucky ones who survived severe botulism. The *Edmonton Bulletin* newspaper reported the strong response to this frightful event:

> "The entire camp supplies where the trouble occurred have been destroyed, including utensils even down to the stove and a complete new outfit installed. The poisoning is said to be a rare of germ known as botilus [sic]. Samples of the blood have been submitted to the most eminent bacteriologists of the North American continent for analysis."

One Victim's Account of Surviving Botulism

Dr. Glancy was able to chronicle his botulism symptoms and personal experience as his case progressed. What follows is an abbreviated version from his thesis on botulism:

"Account of my own illness: I found that there was a certain haziness over my eyes; this condition lasted for about half an hour and passed away.

I had dinner at 6:00 p.m. and about half an hour after dinner I felt the haziness of vision returning. At 8:30 p.m. I walked the distance of about five good city blocks. I noticed that the haziness of vision was still present to the same degree but that added to this was an uncertainty of step, a feeling that I was stepping high and 'walking on air'.

I attended a dance that evening [Saturday] and noticed that if I remained quiet for long at a time the dimness of vision became greater, whereas while actively on the move I scarcely noticed it. I slept well that night. And added to this was diplopia, which came on for a couple of minutes at varying intervals … Realizing that I was getting weaker very rapidly, I called for a car and was taken to the hospital as a patient.

Every symptom so far mentioned seemed to be increasing in severity and along with this, extreme muscular weakness. . . . The following day I noticed that my eyelids were drooping slightly, my pupils were dilated and diplopia was

"more marked. Was very restless, and
perspired a great deal. I began at
this time to have some difficulty in
swallowing."

At this point, five men in the camp were sent to Dawson City with symptoms of hazy vision and disturbed gait, meaning they walked as if intoxicated. They were under the medical treatment of Dr. Glancy, who also showed mild symptoms of poisoning. Dr. Glancy had difficulty walking and vision disturbances, but he still attended a dance four days after the meal in question. He was actively moving at the dance. He even slept well that night. However, the day after, he had double vision and admitted himself to the hospital, giving charge of his patients to Dr. Culbertson and Dr. LaChapelle.

Six days after ingestion of botulinum toxin, while in St. Mary's hospital in Dawson City, Dr. Glancy's symptoms intensified.

"By Tuesday my throat, particularly
the right side of the soft palate,
pharynx, and uvula, seemed paralyzed.
I could scarcely swallow at all and my
voice, was reduced to a whisper. My
throat became clogged with a thick,
glairy, tenacious mucous which I had
great difficulty in expelling. My
tongue was becoming thick posteriorly
at this time. The weakness of my
muscles in general was becoming such
that I found it an effort to move my
limbs in bed. I noticed that my right
arm was weaker than my left, though
normally it is the reverse."

In the following couple of days the above mentioned symptoms all became more severe, it was almost impossible to raise my right hand to my head, I could get my left there with much less difficulty. The extensor muscles of my forearm and hand were particularly affected, also the supinators and pronators of the hand, the flexors were not affected proportionately."

Dr. Glancy continued to note some unusual manifestations of the classic botulism symptoms; he documented the asymmetrical quality to his flaccid paralysis. Such atypical manifestations are often lost in the generalized diagnostic guidelines used in modern medicine today. Paralysis is usually–but not always–symmetrical in botulism cases, thus one-sided paralysis can lead to modern physicians dismissing botulism as a possible diagnosis. Dr. Glancy recorded minute details:

"Of the fingers the middle and ring fingers were affected most, I am referring here to the right hand and arm. The left side was weak, but the muscles affected were not marked off so distinctly in groups. My tongue now had a thick grayish-black coating and my breath was very bad.

Any difficulty I had up to this time in relation to breathing seemed to be a result of the respiratory mechanism. I could see no expansion of the chest at all and it seemed like to be a result of the mucous, now, there was added to this, extreme muscular weakness and a paralysis, I believe, of the respiratory mechanism. I could

see no expansion of the chest at all
and it seemed like a leaden weight."

This "leaden weight" Dr. Glancy describes is the distress often felt by a patient prior to respiratory collapse. The patient has the will to breathe, but has no control over the physical ability to inhale. The diaphragm muscles do not receive the signal from the nerves to contract because of the damage by botulinum toxin. The 'leaden weight' is a horrifying sensation likened to suffocation.

Dr. Glancy documented his symptoms as his condition worsened:

"It was at this time in my illness
that I had a period of about twelve
hours in which my condition, from a
respiratory standpoint at least, was
considered the worst. My pulse was of
very small volume but regular in
rhythm, the rate varied from 88 to
100, my usual rate being 80. My
temperature remained normal throughout
this bad spell.

Following this I perspired freely and
was able to breathe more easily. About
twelve hours later I had a similar
attack but not quite as severe, the
whole condition of general weakness,
excessive mucous in the throat,
difficult breathing and weakened heart
prevailed as in the former one,
however.

The only other new symptom following
this, up to the time that I noticed an
improvement in my condition, was a
severe left sided headache."

Another atypical symptom–yet common in reports on botulinum toxin poisoning–is a severe headache. Botulism induces not just mild headaches, but severe headaches that patients find difficult to describe using traditional pain scales.

"On the eighteenth day in hospital, a dull pain came on in the aortic and pulmonary areas, this continued present to the same degree until June 22, which was the first time that I got a really noticeable expansion of my chest, until now my breathing had been all abdominal and that limited. Up to this time I had lost twenty pounds."

Within one month of being poisoned by botulinum toxin, Dr. Glancy had lost twenty pounds, unable to swallow adequate nourishment. He was fortunate that his cardiac issues did not lead to a fatality, as so often is seen in botulism illnesses.

"From this time on there was a very gradual improvement in every way, and I left the hospital on July 5th to recuperate at a friend's home. By the last of July the pain in the pulmonary and aortic areas had practically gone, I still had some ptosis and lack of expression, was also very easily tired and required to walk with a cane all the time."

Dr. Glancy was hospitalized for forty days– from May 26 to July 5, 1919. Two months later, in September, while still recovering and walking with a cane, he traveled from the Yukon Territory to San Francisco, California. Dr. E.C. Dickson, a professor at Stanford University, examined Dr. Glancy. Dickson had published a lengthy monograph on botulism in 1918 with funding from the Rockefeller Institute for Medical Research.

Dr. Glancy published the symptoms of botulism he witnessed in this large botulism outbreak:

- Haziness of vision that would come and go
- Constipation
- Difficulty walking with coordination
- Double vision
- Ebb and flow of symptoms
- Perspiration and restlessness
- Extreme fatigue
- Generalized muscle weakness
- Inability to walk
- Arms weaker than legs
- Lack of facial expression
- Swollen eyelids (ptosis)
- Difficulty swallowing
- Voice reduced to a whisper
- Mucus in throat
- Swollen tongue
- Slurred speech
- Difficulty breathing
- Unable to inflate lungs
- Feeling of extreme suffocation for long periods
- Weakened heart
- Severe headache
- Asymmetric flaccid paralysis
- Pins and needles sensation in the fingertips
- Good and bad periods
- Control of mental faculties throughout

Six months after botulism, Dr. Glancy's own health status was improving. His arm strength had returned. He tired easily and frequently. Haziness of vision was still present when he was overly tired, but the vision issues were intermittent. He experienced shortness of breath upon exertion. The local newspaper reported that he was "lacking his old-time vigor." Eleven months post-botulism, Dr. Glancy was symptom-free except for a slight tremor of the hands. He had gained back all but four pounds of the weight he had lost during his hospitalization. After his recovery, he accepted a position at St. Anthony's Hospital in Toronto. He married Violet Jones who bore their son, Kenneth, in 1926. Kenneth's son possesses his grandfather's diary from his time in Dawson City.

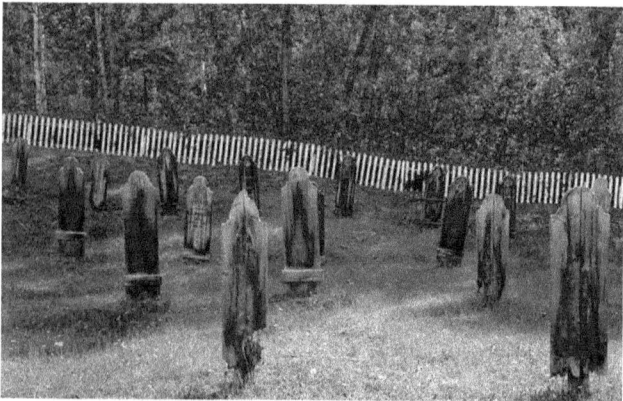

Yukon Order of Pioneers Cemetery, Dawson City

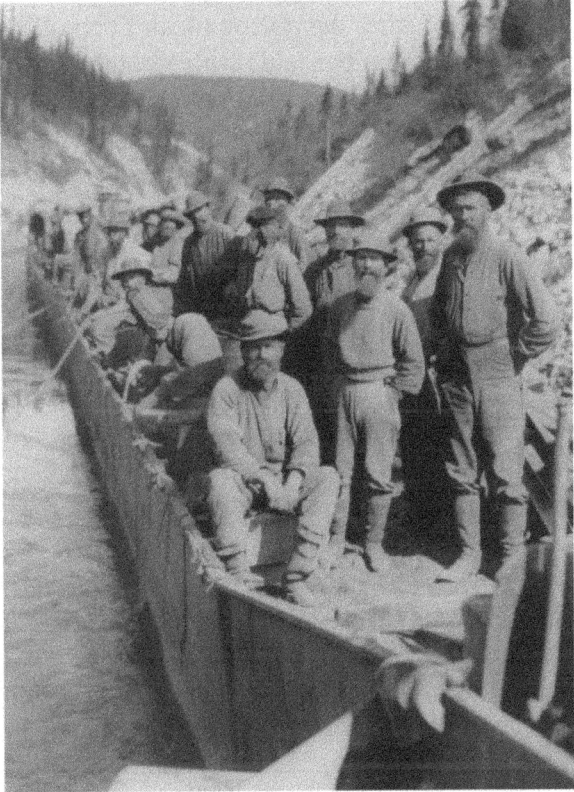

The Twelve Fatalities

The Klondike Gold Rush of 1896 attracted one hundred thousand fortune seekers from all over the world, but most of them could not bear the conditions. Many would-be gold prospectors became entrepreneurs to serve the miners. The Yukon Order of Pioneers cemetery is the final resting place for several of the victims from the botulism outbreak at the gold mining camp.

All twelve fatalities occurred within six to eleven days after the poison meal. Each of the four widows was compensated with $2,500 for the death of her husband from the Yukon Gold Company. The fifth widow was compensated with $1,000 because her husband was not an employee of Yukon Gold Company, but was a boarder in the mess house.

1

Alphonse Rioux, age forty-four, was a native of Montreal. His earliest symptom was vomiting. He then had a great pain in the back of his head, was unable to speak, had difficulty swallowing, and had generalized weakness. Then came death. He left behind a daughter.

2

John Grant, age fifty-three, was a native of Antigonish, Nova Scotia. He was prominent in silver mining at Aspen, Colorado, where he was also sheriff. He was the brother-in-law of the man credited with the co-discovery of gold in the Klondike, Rob Henderson. Initially, John felt intoxicated and his speech was indistinct from having a thick tongue. He could not swallow. He suffered general weakness, restlessness, pain in the head, and tightness in the chest. His death came after his sudden collapse. He left behind a wife and eight children in Dawson.

3

John William McNeill, age unknown, was a native of Antigonish, Nova Scotia. He had a tottering gait and vision disturbances. He was unable to swallow and had impaired speech. His right arm was paralyzed, but not his left. He experienced a sense of suffocation. Then came death.

4

John Thompson, age forty-nine, was a native of Ireland. He was very ill, had numb arms, and was unable to swallow. Then came death.

5

Adrian Barrett, age forty, was a native of Bartholomew, Quebec. He was weak, scarcely able to talk, and was unable to swallow. After three weak spells. Then came death.

6

William Cyrus Lawson, age thirty-nine, was a native of Fort Scott, Kansas, and formerly a prominent dredge man of Oroville, California. Lawson was the assistant superintendent of the Yukon Gold Company of Dawson. He vomited, had difficulty walking, impaired vision, double vision, and was dizzy and weak. He had tightness of the chest. Then came death. He left behind a wife in Dawson and a son in the Aviation Corps in France.

7

Albert Gaudreau, age forty-nine, was a native of St. Thomas, Quebec. Early symptoms were a haziness of vision and double vision. He had no muscular weakness. On May 24, two days after the meal, he "laughed at the idea of going to bed." By May 26, his speech was impaired and he was restless. On May 27, he had a great deal of pain in his head. Then came death.

8

Angus Chisholm, age forty, was a native of Antigonish, Nova Scotia. Early symptoms were a haziness of vision and double vision. He took a bath without assistance and went to bed. He felt better the next day, but by evening he became weaker. His arms went numb and he reported a great deal of pain along his spinal cord prior to his death. He left behind a wife and two small children in Vancouver, Canada.

9

Finley McDonald, age sixty-two, was from New Glasgow, Nova Scotia. Initial symptoms included slight double vision and a mild headache. He took a bath without assistance, walked easily down the hall, and was in good spirits. In a couple of days, he developed difficulty swallowing and speaking. He complained of a very severe pain in the head and perspired greatly. Pulse was 140 just before death.

10

Otto Nordling, age forty-eight, was a native of Sweden. His condition was not serious because he had only some nausea and no difficulty in speech or swallowing. Two days later, he had a sore throat and difficulty swallowing. Then came severe pains in the occipital region and his spinal cord. He was restless prior to his death. He left behind a wife and five children in Dawson.

11

George Mundeen, age forty-three, was a native of Montreal. He had slightly impaired speech. He indulged freely of liquor when he realized he had ingested poison, thinking it would be beneficial, but due to his alcohol intoxication the diagnosis was delayed. He was very restless, had respiratory distress, and then died.

12

Antoine Zadielovich, age unknown, was a native of Dalmatia (now Austria-Hungary). He was a waiter at the camp. He refused to go to the hospital until authorities compelled him to seek medical attention. He had impaired speech, difficulty swallowing, and respiratory difficulties. His pulse was 130 at death.

Dr. Glancy put forth enormous effort to gather the details of those who survived the botulism outbreak. Recall, he was still in the throes of recovery himself for most of 1919 when this research was conducted.

Seven Other Individuals Who Recovered

1

Mr. O. C., age twenty-five, vomited half an hour after the meal. The next day he felt weak and had some blurry vision. A few days later his tongue was dry, hard, and rough. It was slightly swollen. His right eyelid was swollen and he had difficulty swallowing. Both arms were weak, but the right arm was weaker. He was easily fatigued with the slightest effort. He was on a fluid diet for five days, then a soft diet for five days, then could tolerate a regular diet by the tenth day. He lost twelve pounds during this illness. The extensor muscles of the forearm and hands were the weakest. Recovery was marked by particularly good days, but then relapsed back to almost his former condition. Because of these continuous relapses, improvement was very gradual. One year later, his arms had not regained their former strength, but were improving gradually. The good periods lasted longer, and while the bad periods of relapses still appeared intermittently, he felt he was making progress.

2

Chris Tomich, age thirty-one, reported that his stomach felt like a stone after the Victoria Day meal. He had blurry vision when he entered the hospital the next day. His tongue was hard, dry, and thick. He expelled thick mucus. His eyes became glassy and the right eyelid swelled shut. Lifting his head off the pillow was difficult; the neck muscles had become weak. He had pain on the lower right occipital region and back of the neck on the side as well. His right arm was weaker than his left. The right leg was also weaker than the left, but not as noticeable as the arms. He had slight double vision. Occasionally, he felt tightness across the chest, but this was of short duration. He had no respiratory difficulty. He lost sixteen pounds while in the hospital for one month. Six months after the incident, he sent a letter stating he had no permanent issues and had been back to work for three months.

3

Emile Wolfe, age thirty-eight, reported early symptoms as haziness of vision, dizziness, nausea, and occasional double vision. He went to work but was weak and stumbled as if drunk. He had constipation from the onset. He felt there was a band around his throat and chest. His tongue was dry and swollen; he spoke with great difficulty. He experienced a choking sensation. A few days later, a weakness over the back of the neck and shoulder blades occurred. Next, his arms were weak, the right one more so than the left. Within a week, his calf muscles and thighs were lame. He limped because one leg was more paralyzed than the other. He reported a "pins and needles" sensation on the ring finger of his right hand. He lost twenty-four pounds while in the hospital for one month. Six months later he reported no permanent effects, and he was employed doing what he called "fairly heavy work."

4

Eugene Lemieux, age thirty-six, first noticed a frontal headache, then blurred vision, vertigo, and pains in the calf muscles of his legs. After three days, the weakness was noticeable and he had to quit work at the gold mine. On the way to Dawson, he was chilled and had considerable pain along his spinal cord. The pain was also severe in the mastoid regions of his jaw. Over the week, he noticed the weakness was increasing and his gait was unsteady. His tongue had also become thick and speech was indistinct. When he finally admitted himself to the hospital about three weeks after the meal, his extensor muscles of his forearms were greatly affected by weakness. Obstinate constipation persisted. He did not have double vision, but things looked larger than usual. He battled glairy mucous secretions and lost twenty-four pounds during the illness. After two weeks in the hospital, his symptoms had dissipated and he was discharged to home. The following November, he spent two months rehabilitating at Tenakee Hot Springs on Chichagof Island in Southeast Alaska–a place known for the 106-degree sulfur water.

5

Antone Boulay, age forty-three, was blind for a few minutes the day after the meal. He rubbed his eyes vigorously and the sight returned, but remained blurred. The following day he noticed he tired immediately at the least exertion. He had a soreness along the costal margin of the rib cage, and his arms and legs were stiff at the elbows and knees. Three days after the meal, he was admitted to the hospital with a severe headache on one side of his skull. He complained of a smothering sensation. His right leg and left arm were weak. The forearm and hand were the weakest muscles. Though his tongue was swollen, his swallowing was only slightly impaired. He left the hospital with some symptoms, but felt he could function at home. However, once home, he had considerable pain along the whole spine, particularly in the lumbar and interscapular region. He also had difficulty breathing. He returned to the hospital for a week and improved rapidly. He lost six pounds during his ordeal.

6

Hugh McAdams, age sixty-one, experienced diarrhea, blurred vision, and an occipital headache two days after the meal. On the third day, he felt weaker. On the fourth day, he had difficulty swallowing, feeling as though there was an obstruction behind his larynx. His tongue was dry and thick. Haziness of vision and dizziness became more prominent. Both arms were weak, but the right arm in particular was very weak. The forearms and hands were affected the greatest. Pupils were dilated and eyes were glassy. One week after the meal, he went to the hospital. There, the eyelids were swollen shut; the right eyelid was the worst. He had difficulty breathing and complained of a dull continuous pain in the rotator cuff. He lost twenty-three pounds during his illness. Recovery was marked with a period of two or three good days, then a relapse back to almost the former condition. He left the hospital after two months but could not physically return to work until five months post-botulism. He still had shortness of breath, upon exertion and he had not regained his weight. Improvement was steady, and he felt certain he would have no permanent after effects - even though at six months he was only partially recovered.

7

George Crowley, age fifty-one, was dizzy and had blurred vision the day after the meal. He felt intoxicated, but did not stagger. The following day, he had double vision. Soon his throat was weak and speech was thick. He also had weakness in his right hip that affected his gait. His right hand was very weak, and he was not able to raise his arm above his head. His throat was paralyzed, mostly on the right side. His tongue was thick and he had difficulty swallowing.

After a week of growing progressively weaker, he went to the hospital. Eyes were worsening and eyelids were swollen shut. The right eye was affected worse than the left. Constipation was present from the beginning. He had no particular difficulty in breathing at any time. By mid-August the blurred vision and ptosis (drooping eyelids) were practically gone. He was on a fluid diet which was difficult due to swallowing issues. He lost twenty-one pounds during the illness. He had good and bad periods on a regular basis. He was hospitalized for three months, the longest of all the victims. He convalesced at a friend's house from September to January and wrote by letter that he was "as active as ever and that he weighed three pounds more than he ever did." He did not experience permanent aftereffects.

Physicians from San Francisco and the brotherly duo of Drs. Mayo and Mayo were consulted on Yukon Territory outbreak. They agreed upon a diagnosis of botulism due to the neurological disorders associated with botulinum toxin poisoning. The meat was the suspected source of the toxin, though no samples were found or sent to hospitals for laboratory confirmation. It is unknown if the illness was caused by botulinum toxin A or botulinum toxin type B.

TAKEAWAYS from
THE YUKON TERRITORY

Paralysis can be asymmetrical in botulism cases.

Pain associated with botulism includes severe headaches, chest pain, and back pain.

Recovery is a process of making slow progress and then occasionally relapsing almost to the original condition.

There is variability in the symptoms even within the same botulism outbreak.

Botulism symptoms wax and wane giving hope for recovery, only to suddenly result in a fatal outcome.

The severity of the illness, even in fatal cases, is initially underestimated by patients.

Severity waxes and wanes. Victims have temporary improvements then steep declines in status resulting in fatal outcomes.

Botulism symptoms unfold at a different pace for each patient and can also present with different severities. Even when all cases result in fatal outcomes, the progression varies greatly.

Complete respiratory collapse from botulism can happen with little to no warning, resulting in death within minutes.

Neither severity of symptoms nor early symptom onset are reliable predictors about the recovery potential or the probability of fatality of a botulism patient.

Cardiac-related deaths in botulism are common.

Recovery from botulism can take days, months, or years.

CHAPTER 5

Botulism Diagnosed over the Phone
THE ALLIANCE, OHIO
OUTBREAK of 1919

On Saturday, August 23, 1919, a dinner and dance were held to celebrate the homecoming of Colonel Charles C. Weybrecht. Over two hundred people gathered at the Lakeside Country Club in Canton, Ohio, to celebrate the Colonel's triumphant return from the battlefields of France. One month earlier, the Colonel had completed his service in the Great War; his hometown welcomed him back with a grand celebration, where he was recognized for his valor in the Spanish-American War, the Mexican Border War, and the Great War.

Unfortunately, no amount of valor on the battlefield would save Colonel Weybrecht from the effects of botulinum toxin in a jar of ripe black olives served to the head table. In less than one week, seven guests, including the Colonel, would be dead. Seven more suffered illness from the poisoning, but would eventually recover to greater or lesser degrees. This celebration would ultimately become known as "The Death Banquet."

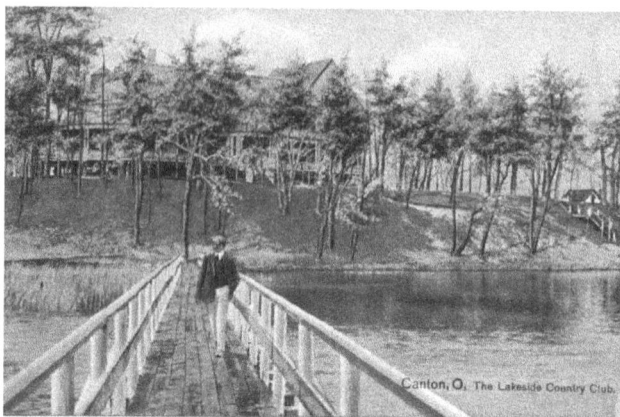

Postcard of The Lakeside Country Club, Canton, Ohio

Rumors would swirl around the event. Some speculated that the poisonings might have been an assassination attempt on the guest of honor, likely perpetrated by the Germans. Then the turkey meat was suspected of contamination. The "demon rum," served by the host, Willard Gahris, despite Prohibition having gone into effect July 1, 1919, was also heavily suspect. The state conducted an extensive epidemiologic investigation that determined the true source of the toxin and laid the rumor mill to rest.

Bill Gahris and Helen Sebring Gahris hosted the celebration, and seated the guest of honor at their table. Helen, an heir to the Sebring Pottery factory, was out to impress. A special effort was made to adorn the Sebring table with exceptional treats: candied almonds, chocolate candy, Newport Creams, and ripe black olives. The other tables at the banquet served more common hors d'oeuvres that included green olives, celery, and pickles.

Helen made a special trip to L.M. Barth grocery to purchase a glass jar of Mammoth Ripe Olives packed by the Curtis Corporation in California. When she handed the olives to the waiter, he opened the jar and placed the olives into three bowls. Two of the bowls of olives he rinsed with water and drained with his fingers. The olives in the third bowl were not rinsed.

There were eighteen guests seated at the Sebring table. Five of the guests, Colonel Charles Weybrecht, Katherine Sharer, John Sharer, Helen Gahris, and Jessie Sanford, as well as two members of the staff–Bob Jennings, a waiter, and Frank McAvoy, the chef–died from botulism. Other guests at the Sebring table survived: the waiter Charles Otey, Emily Weybrecht, Louis Busch, Maude Busch, Clem Bates, Mary Bates, William Morgan, and Annette Morgan all developed very mild symptoms of botulism, but later recovered.

Initially, the people who became ill all sought medical attention from different physicians and all were misdiagnosed. The first to die was Robert Jennings, a black waiter at Lakeside Country Club. He vomited twenty-six hours after the meal. His symptoms included double vision, weakness, and difficulty of speech. Surprisingly, he had no ptosis of the eyelids. Robert Paul Jennings, age thirty-four, died on Monday afternoon just fifty-four hours after he ate six olives.

Chef Frank McAvoy experienced ptosis in both eyelids. He also had dimness of vision, double vision, thirst, weakness, difficulty of speech, dizziness, vomiting, constipation, loss of voice, and difficulty swallowing. Frank D. McAvoy, age sixty-five, died at 9:00 AM Wednesday, seventy-five hours after eating just two olives. Both employees sought medical attention from the house physician for the club, Dr. J.P. DeWitt.

Chef Who Cooked Dinner Also Dead

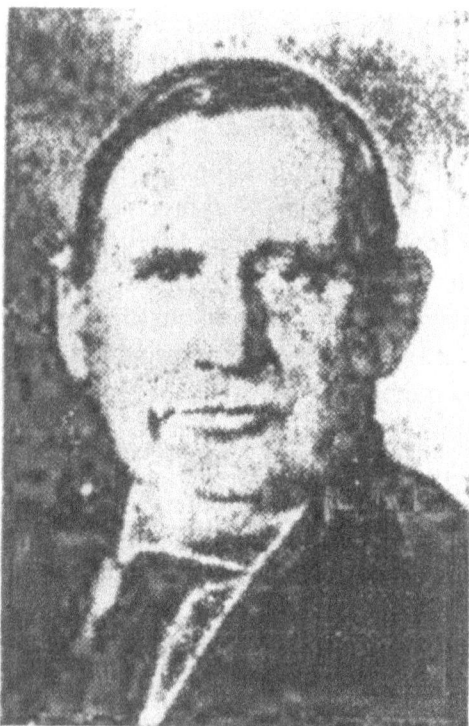

Frank D. McAvoy

Colonel Weybrecht became nauseated immediately after dinner on Saturday night. He vomited four hours later that evening. His first neurological symptom was Sunday when he experienced vision issues on a walk with his brother

Ben. Later that day, during an automobile ride with Ben, the Colonel saw two objects when there was just one. He remarked that he probably needed eyeglasses. His symptoms progressed the following day. He had dim vision, difficulty of speech, weakness, and loss of voice. Surprisingly, he also did not have ptosis in either eyelid. His was the only fatal case to have paresthesia, a tingling burning sensation described as "pins and needles." Early in the illness Colonel Weybrecht's family physician, Dr. Hoover, attributed his condition to a cerebral hemorrhage.

William Morgan and his brother-in-law John Sharer and John's wife Kit went mushroom hunting the Sunday morning after the dinner. When John's symptoms developed, he initially assumed that the mushrooms they had foraged and prepared for dinner that night to be at fault. Those symptoms began on Monday when John visited his mother and his father (General John Sharer) at their home. As John looked out the window, he asked his mother whether she saw two girls walking up Union Avenue; he thought it was odd that they were dressed alike and moving in unison. When John's mother assured him there was only one girl, John commented that he had better get his eyes checked.

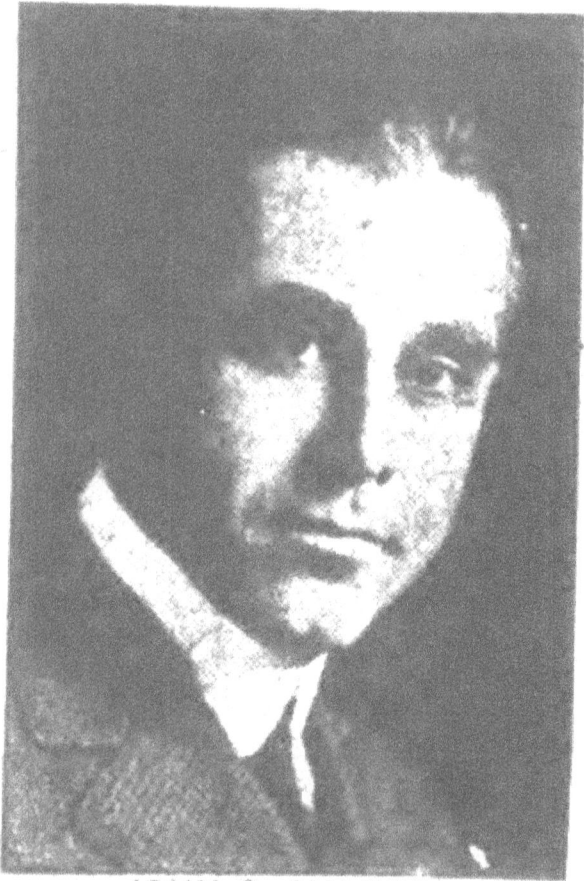

JOHN C. SHARER

John Sharer

Once back home, John and his wife, Katherine (Kit), experienced more symptoms. Their speech, swallowing, and breathing were impaired. Their family physician, Dr. John Roach, came by their house early in the illness and suspected they had fungus poisoning from eating freshly picked puff balls. Nurses were called to stay with the Sharers all day. John developed abdominal pain and thick mucus in his throat. He also experienced thirst, double vision, dim vision, difficulty of speech, dizziness, vomiting, constipation, and ptosis in both eyelids. Kit had all the same symptoms plus a slight headache. She vomited after being given a dose of castor oil. Neither John nor Kit lost their voices.

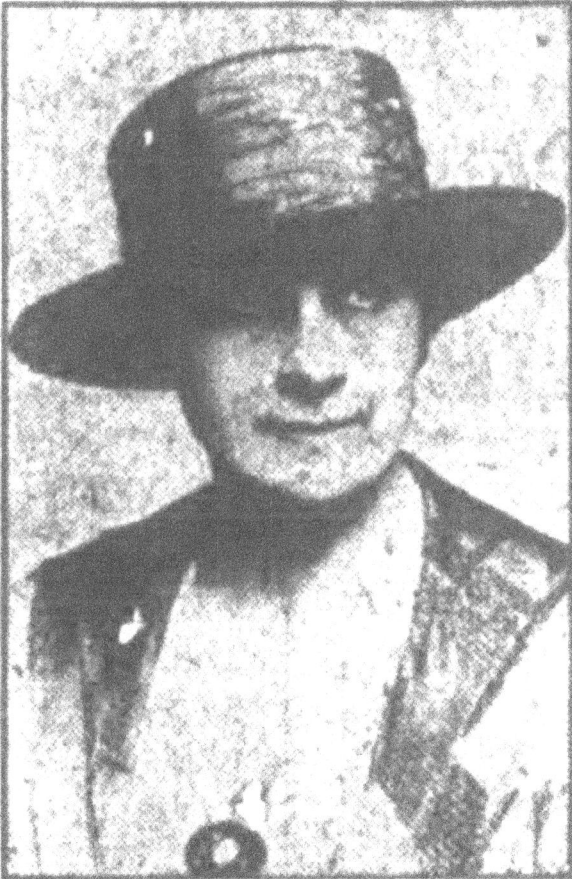

MRS. JOHN C. SHARER
Kit Sharer

William Morgan was thunderstruck when he was told about the illnesses. He felt that he was responsible, and must have made a mistake in his identification of the edible mushrooms and poison puffballs. Later that same afternoon, Ben Weybrecht, brother of the guest of honor Colonel Weybrecht, called William to tell him that the Colonel was very ill and that the doctor thought that Colonel Weybrecht had suffered a cerebral hemorrhage. William was naturally distressed, but at that time there seemed no connection between the Sharers' illnesses and Colonel Weybrecht's health issue.

Around dinner time, William received word that Helen Gahris was also very ill, and that her doctor thought that she had contracted ptomaine poisoning. It was William Morgan who made the connection. He reasoned that the illnesses were all the same, and that whatever caused the maladies would have to be related to the previous Saturday night when the victims were all at the same dinner party, eating at the same table.

William immediately called Dr. Roach, told him of his conclusion, and suggested that he contact the other doctors involved. Dr. Roach called back shortly and reported that the doctors had conferred and agreed that all of the victims had been poisoned, but did not know what kind of poison it was. They felt that the foremost authority in this area was Dr. John Phillips in Cleveland. (He was the future co-founder of the famed Cleveland Clinic.) Dr. Phillips was reached by telephone at 9:00 PM on Monday evening.

Upon hearing about the symptoms, Dr. Phillips said that he was almost sure these were cases of botulism. He had never seen a case of botulism, but had recently read a medical article about it. Even over the phone, Dr. Phillips was versed enough in botulism symptoms to recognize the disease and make a diagnosis sight unseen. He was extremely interested in the outbreak and left Cleveland immediately by car for Alliance, Ohio.

When Dr. Phillips arrived at midnight, he found the Colonel in critical condition. A physical examination confirmed Dr. Phillips's suspicions of botulism. Colonel Weybrecht was unable to speak, but was able to write a question on a pad of paper, "What are my chances?" Dr. Phillips reassured him, but the Colonel had his own conclusions in reply as he scrawled "50-50" on paper.

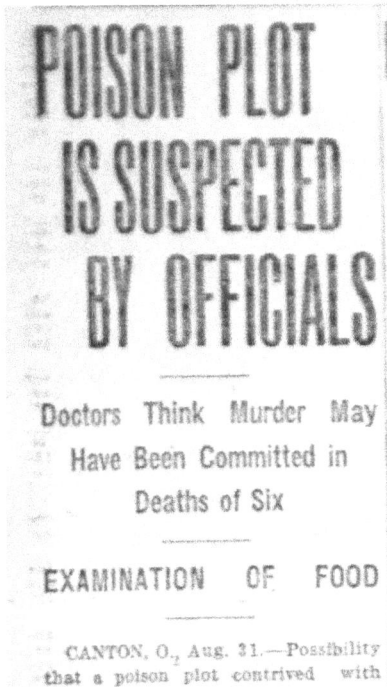

POISON PLOT IS SUSPECTED BY OFFICIALS

Doctors Think Murder May Have Been Committed in Deaths of Six

EXAMINATION OF FOOD

CANTON, O., Aug. 31.—Possibility that a poison plot contrived with

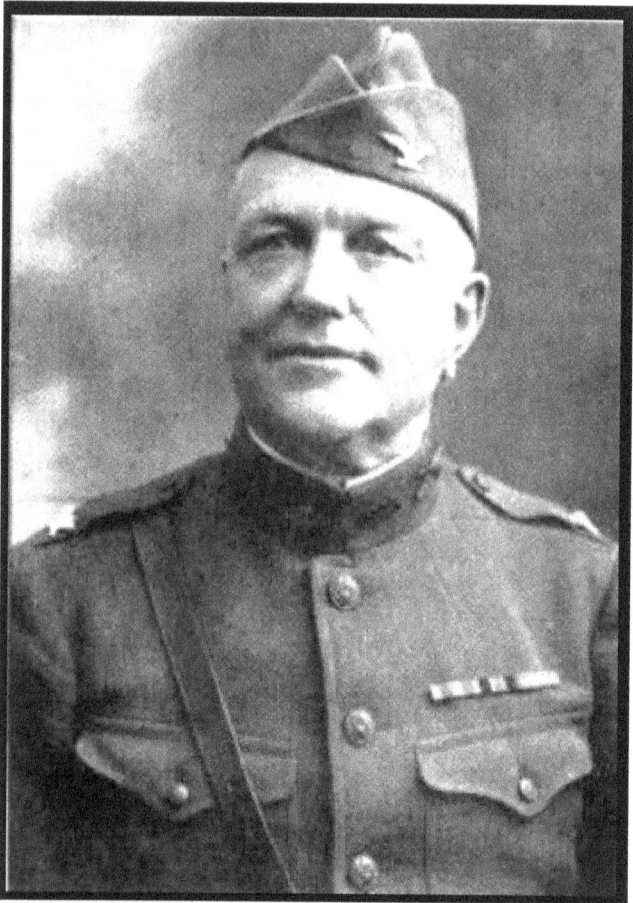

Colonel Charles C. Weybrecht

Colonel Charles C. Weybrecht, age fifty-one, died at 4:00 AM Tuesday morning. Later that week, the funeral procession for Col. Weybrecht in Alliance, Ohio, population twenty thousand, was ten blocks long and drew a crowd of ten thousand people. The mayor requested that all businesses and shops be closed that day to celebrate the town's "favorite son." The funeral procession included a military presence consisting of a firing squad from Company K, Company B, and the 146th U.S. Infantry, Great War veterans, Spanish American War veterans, and veterans of the Army, Navy, and Marines. The 146th Infantry Band of Akron led the military division. After the death of her husband, Emily Weybrecht, one of the victims who made a recovery, moved to Seward, Alaska, to live with her brother, Cal Brosius.

Helen Gahris played golf on Sunday following the banquet celebration and complained of double vision. By Monday, she was suffering from dimness of vision, weakness, difficulty swallowing, and ptosis in both eyelids. She also lost her voice. Her physician initially ascribed her sickness to ptomaine poisoning. Dr. Phillips planned to drive to nearby Sebring, Ohio, to see Helen on Tuesday, but a telephone call brought the sad news that Helen Sebring Gahris, age thirty-three, had died at 3:00 AM Tuesday morning. She left behind her husband Bill and their daughter, Gretchen, age seven.

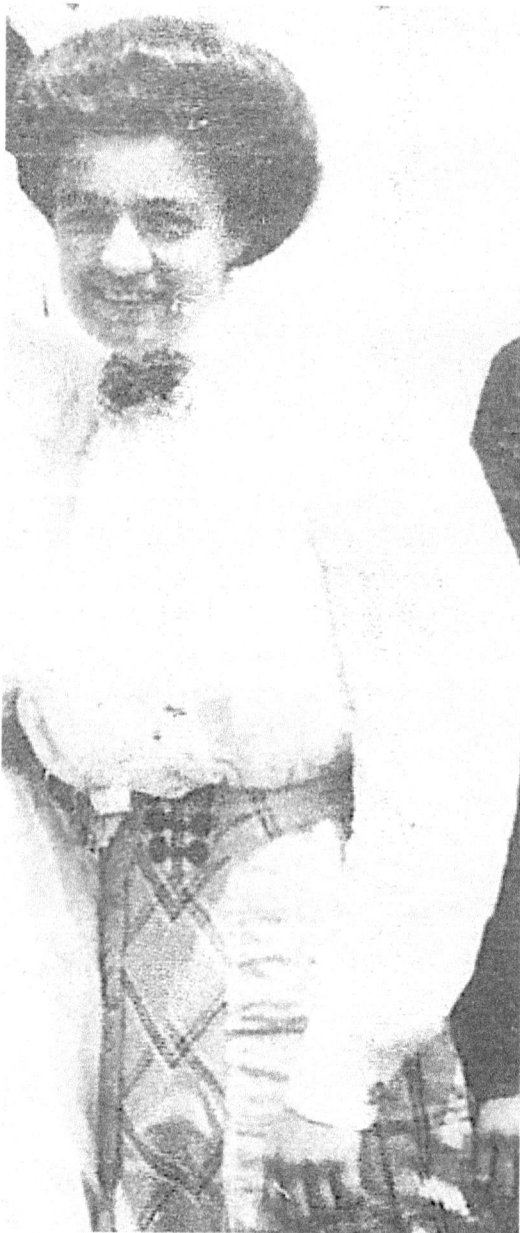

Helen Gahris

Dr. Phillips went to the Sharer home on Tuesday, and his diagnoses of botulism were further confirmed by examining the Sharers. John Sharer, age forty-nine, died of botulism at 5:15 PM Tuesday evening; Kit, age thirty-nine, died at 10:30 AM on Wednesday morning.

The last fatal case was Jessie Sanford, the wife of Willis Sanford, a local dentist. Jessie and Willis had two children—Susan, age three, and William, age eighteen months. Jessie distinctly recalled biting into an olive and not liking the taste. She swallowed half of the olive and set the remainder aside.

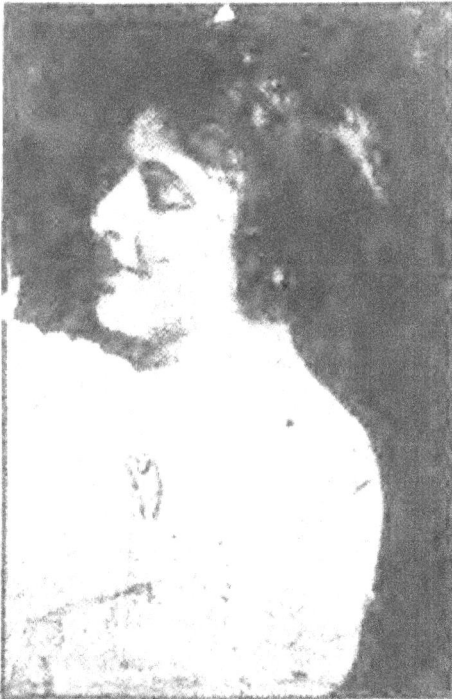

MRS. WILLIS F. SANFORD

Jessie Sanford

Jessie's physician, Dr. L.F. Mutschmann, reported her symptoms two days after the meal as slight headache, double vision, moderate dimness of vision, and a very slight vertigo. Jessie's pupil reflexes were sluggish. She had ptosis in the left eyelid only, and she had a "partial inability to rotate her left eye externally." The mucus membranes in her throat and nose were moderately congested. There was no change in speech. The heart gave a "slightly accentuated second sound."

On the third day after the meal, Jessie had trouble swallowing. The vertigo and headache persisted. Her temperature, pulse, and respiration remained unchanged. She was able to take some nutrition and was fairly comfortable despite showing symptoms of botulism. That evening, swallowing and speech became more difficult.

On the fourth day, Jessie was able to gargle, but unable to swallow. She complained of a slight pain and a "distressing burning sensation" in the abdomen. The colicky pains in the lower abdomen resolved after she had a bowel movement. By 9:00 PM on the fourth day, she was greatly distressed by pain and constriction of the throat.

The information about the other six deaths was withheld from Jessie for fear the bad news would negatively impact how hard she fought the illness. She kept insisting that her husband go back to work at his dental office and expressed surprise that he remained at home during her illness.

On the morning of the fifth day, Jessie remained in the same condition except she was drowsy and had a dry throat. She could not protrude her tongue past her lips. At 7:00 PM she was "relieved quite suddenly of the dryness in the throat and mouth and was able to move her tongue more freely," prompting her to try to take liquids. However, she could not swallow. The waxing and waning of symptoms is a common occurrence as botulism progresses. At 10:00 PM, Jessie complained of pain in the region of the heart that traveled through the left axilla to her back, where it lasted for five minutes. During this time, she experienced "slight difficulty in breathing and became very restless."

On the sixth day, Jessie's throat was once again very dry and raw; she had the sensation that her throat was closing up. She was extremely weak. Though she was able to sleep for short intervals, she awoke to an alarming choking sensation that was coupled with turning blue in the face. That night, she was extremely fatigued but slept only for one hour in total. As a last-ditch effort, she was given two injections of the experimental botulism antitoxin developed by Dr. Robert Graham at the University of Illinois in Champaign, Illinois. After each injection, Jessie perspired profusely and complained of feeling hot and very tired. However, within an hour, she reported that she felt improved.

On the seventh day, Jessie's pulse increased to 118. Her body felt cold and clammy. Respirations were shallow and slightly irregular. Her pulse hit 126 and the coloring of her skin was quite blue, but Jessie appeared to be weak and resting.

On her eighth and last day in this world, Jessie's pulse was 158. She was too weak to move in bed and had lost the ability to speak. The cyanosis spread; she was blue all over her body. Her perspirations were profuse and cold. Her respiration ceased and cardiac failure occurred.

Jessie Williams Sanford, age thirty-three, passed away on August 30, one week after the meal.

Commonalities of the Fatal Cases

Of the seven fatal cases, four symptoms were present in everyone: double vision, weakness, difficulty swallowing, and difficulty of speech. Six out of seven reported a dimness of vision and dizziness. Five out of seven experienced vomiting. Only one person reported a headache. Only two fatal cases were constipated from paralyzed bowels. About half of the fatalities also suffered extreme thirst, loss of voice, pain, and ptosis of the eyelids.

The Survivors

Charles Otey, a black waiter at the banquet, age thirty-three, was reported to have eaten two olives after the event. He noticed they didn't taste right and asked the chef to sample the offensive olives. Charles said, "try one of these damn things, they don't taste right to me." Olives were a fairly new delicacy, so the chef sampled one, then subsequently died of botulism a few days later.

Charles became "desperately ill" with botulism and was admitted to the hospital in Canton, but eventually recovered. He had consumed a considerable amount of whiskey both before and after eating the olives, which may have contributed to his survival. Ten days after the meal, his status was reported as "somewhat improved his vision however is still affected."

Emily Weybrecht had mild symptoms of botulism that resolved. She had a headache, double vision, difficulty of speech, constipation, and two atypical symptoms of botulism–paresthesia (pins and needles sensation) and hyperesthesia, an increased sensitivity, which in Emily's case manifested as a sensitivity to light.

Louis Busch, the publisher of the *Salem News* and *East Liverpool Review* newspapers, had double vision from August through mid-September. Early on he had a headache, dimness of vision, dizziness, difficulty swallowing, and a slight case of hyperesthesia. Noticeably absent was any complaint of weakness. His wife, Maude Busch, was also poisoned, and the more seriously ill of the pair. Her symptoms included headache, dimness of vision, difficulty of speech, dizziness, and ptosis of both eyelids. Ten days after the meal, the newspaper reported that they had "considerable trouble with their eyes but had not developed any symptoms of throat paralysis." During the dinner, Maude noticed a black spot on the olive and washed it in some water before eating it. Physicians credit this move with saving her life. She lived to the age of seventy-six.

Mary and Clem Bates also developed poisoning symptoms. Mary's symptoms included thirst, a headache, double vision, dimness of vision, difficulty of speech, dizziness, constipation, ptosis of both eyelids, and difficulty swallowing. It was ten days before Mary was able to swallow solid food. Clem Bates did not experience double vision or ptosis of the eyelids or thirst. However, his symptoms did include a dimness of vision, headache, and constipation. He also vomited six times during the first week. Clem also suffered hyperesthesia; in his case, the neuropathy caused severe pain from the slightest touch to his skin. This is caused by nerve damage from botulinum toxin. Sixteen days after the meal, Clem was still profoundly weak, although his paralytic issues of the eyes and throat had resolved.

William Morgan, the man who initially realized all of the illnesses were connected, suffered mild symptoms of weakness, a change in his voice, and a slight difficulty of speech. The serum drawn from him two days after symptom onset contained enough botulinum toxin that proved to be deadly to guinea pigs in a toxicity test used to assess lethality.

Annette, William Morgan's wife, noted her olive was soft, and not black as it should have been; it had a mottled brown appearance. She took one bite, and since it did not taste right, put it down and did not touch it again. Annette admitted years later to her son that she was very ill the week following the dinner. Fifty years later in an oral history recollection about the tragedy, the grown son reported that during the outbreak his mother's "eyes did not focus properly, and she felt generally bad, but simply had to keep going." Annette Morgan's eyesight was excellent prior to having botulism and was never as good after she recovered from what was considered a very mild case of botulism.

Fred and Ella Morris, who were also present at the Colonel's table during the infamous banquet, did not experience botulism symptoms because they did not eat any olives that evening. Ella thought that the olive she had taken did not smell right, and cautioned her husband, Fred to not eat any. Fortunately for him, he heeded her advice. (While botulinum toxin has no taste or smell, the food product itself can still become degraded.)

Commonalities of the Surviving Cases

For those who recovered, the most common symptoms were dimness of vision, weakness, difficulty of speech, and constipation. It is notable that two of the survivors reported no muscle weakness even though they were severely ill. One survivor in this group suffered paresthesia, a "pins and needles" neuropathy. Four of the seven who recovered experienced hyperesthesia, a condition where the slightest sensation to the skin causes great pain. This pain can be from a light physical touch to the skin or from sunlight that hurts the eyes.

The recovery period discussed in the newspapers indicated the people who survived botulism suffered health issues for weeks and months, but no final follow-up was done to assess the degree of recovery or how long the damage from botulism persisted.

After Helen Gahris died, her brother Charles wanted answers. He petitioned the state of Ohio to get involved because there were competing theories about the tragedy, with some wondering whether it was an accidental poisoning or a murderous plot using poison curare, a plant-derived toxin used to make poison darts.

The state officials appointed George Armstrong, MD to serve as the epidemiologist leading the investigation on the Ohio outbreak. By 1919, Dr. Armstrong had already served in the Great War and was working at the Ohio State Department of Health. He was also a native of Alliance and was personally acquainted with many of the guests impacted by the botulism poisoning.

Others worked the outbreak too. The coroner of Stark County, Ohio, ran tests for a month following the deaths and found the liquid from the jar of olives to be lethal to mice and guinea pigs. Chemical analysis was done by J.G. Spencer of Western Reserve in Cleveland, Ohio. Dr. J.P. DeWitt, the house physician at the country club, injected rabbits with liquid from the suspected olives. The rabbits died within twenty-four hours and showed symptoms similar to the human botulism victims.

Dr. George Armstrong took a personal interest in ascertaining the truth, even running additional experiments to better understand the nature of this lethal botulinum toxin. He was curious how long the toxin circulated in the bloodstream of the survivors. (This is a question that continues to intrigue researchers today.) He injected the serum from William Morgan, Clem Bates, and Charles Otey into guinea pigs to test if the patients who recovered from botulism still had toxin circulating in the bloodstream; the guinea pigs died, which proved the toxin persisted in the blood of patients who were recovering from mild botulism. This research used sixty guinea pigs in the quest to develop new research findings on botulism.

Dr. Armstrong and his colleagues published an unusually long thirty-two-page case report. Later in life he would go on to be recognized for his groundbreaking research in polio, another paralytic disease similar to botulism.

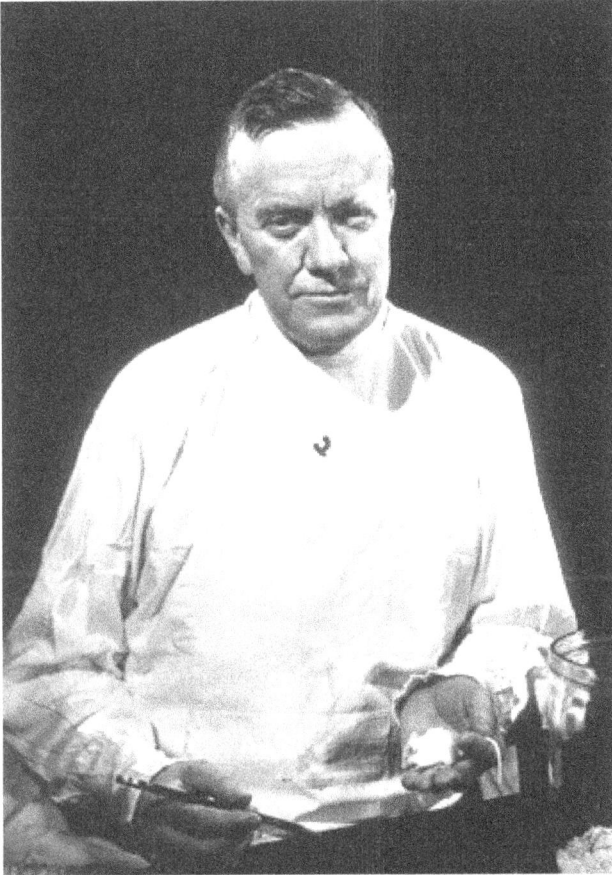

Dr. George Armstrong, MD

After the Ohio and Detroit tragedies, botulism outbreaks continued with disconcerting regularity. A federal regulatory loophole in the 1906 Pure Food and Drugs Act hindered the federal government from acting swiftly regarding the safety of canned goods, and the only immediate remedy fell upon the state health officials.

TAKEAWAYS from
THE OHIO OUTBREAK

Misdiagnosis is common when each patient presents as a solitary case.

There can be variability in the symptoms even within the same botulism outbreak.

Within a single botulism outbreak, patients can share some symptoms in common but also present combinations different from one another.

A physician versed in the clinical symptoms of botulism can make an accurate diagnosis even without seeing the patient.

Botulism presents a distinct set of neurological symptoms that can easily be misdiagnosed when the treating physician lacks direct experience with botulism.

The guinea pigs that were injected with liquids containing trace amounts of botulinum toxin died of botulism.

Botulism patients often underestimate their condition's severity; sudden decline and death can surprise both patient and physician.

Severity waxes and wanes. Victims have temporary improvements then steep declines in status, resulting in fatal outcomes.

Complete respiratory collapse from botulism can happen with little to no warning, resulting in death within minutes.

Neither severity of symptoms nor early symptom onset are reliable predictors about the recovery potential or the probability of fatality of a botulism patient.

CHAPTER 6

The Slow Death Spiral of Botulism
THE HOMEBREW
OUTBREAK of 1919

In the fall of 1919, six men gathered for a BBQ and poker game at the Triplett Ranch located on Stony Creek near Stonyford, California. In January of 1919, the Eighteenth Amendment of the U.S. Constitution was ratified by thirty-six states making alcohol production and recreational alcohol consumption illegal. Two of the men at the ranch took it upon themselves to provide alcohol of their own making for the gathering. The homebrew would become the cause of a botulism outbreak affecting all of the men present. Two survived. Two died within a week. Two lingered for weeks before succumbing to the poison.

Stressors were ample in the United States in 1919. The Great War ended in 1918, but the troops that came home alive continued to battle shell shock (the historical precursor to the later diagnosis of PTSD, post-traumatic stress syndrome) and depression once home. The Great Influenza epidemic followed closely on its heels, claiming the lives of millions with waves of illness in both 1918 and 1919. In the midst of the collective stress of the times, laws passed that made recreational alcohol illegal, sparking a wave of bootlegging operations that produced alcohol for distribution to organized crime rings. To satisfy demand for personal consumption, determined individuals dabbled in homebrewing and building moonshine stills. Occasionally, their concoctions were deadly.

Frank Carney and Andrew Jackson "Jack" Triplett were the brewers of an unfortunate concoction, prepared for the weekend BBQ event, and it was with the best of intentions that they shared their homebrewed wine with four friends: Chas Anderson, Denny O'Leary, Andy O'Leary, and Cash Martin.

Frank and Jack lived on the Triplett Ranch, a 400-acre farm on Stony Creek in Colusa County about seventy miles northwest of Yuba City, California. Frank, age fifty-nine, was a native of Sheboygan, Wisconsin, who had been a widower for many years. He was well-known in the county due to his work on the ranches. Jack, age forty-four, was a native of nearby Maxwell, California. He also rented five acres from his brother, Abraham Lincoln Triplett, to raise watermelons and tomatoes on a commercial scale.

The columnists and readers in the local newspapers maintained a good-natured banter about the water in Stony Creek having medicinal benefits and even magical healing properties. Sometimes they referred to Stony Creek's water as having a *kick* to it because of the illicit alcohol production in the area. The *Alturas New Era* newspaper reported:

> "It appears the men took several cans each of peaches, tomatoes, apricots and grapes and poured them all into a barrel of water, letting it remain until fermentation took place. It had a kick all right, but it kicked and kept kicking until two were dead and two others are at death's door. One can of tomatoes was said to have been seven years old."

The local news reported that Frank and Jack "sampled their mixture on Thursday, September 11, and found it so satisfactory that they decided to have in several of their friends for a little poker game to pass judgment on the drink before the big barbecue." The poker game was held on Saturday, September 13, and a large quantity of wine was consumed.

That Sunday, September 14, Frank and Jack were both quite ill; Dr. W.T. Rathbun was called. Both had paralyzed throats and vision disturbances. They were hospitalized later that week in Colusa.

Denny O'Leary's illness was brief because his wife had "taken him to task" when he arrived home Sunday morning. She gave Denny large doses of 'physic' medicine to make him vomit.

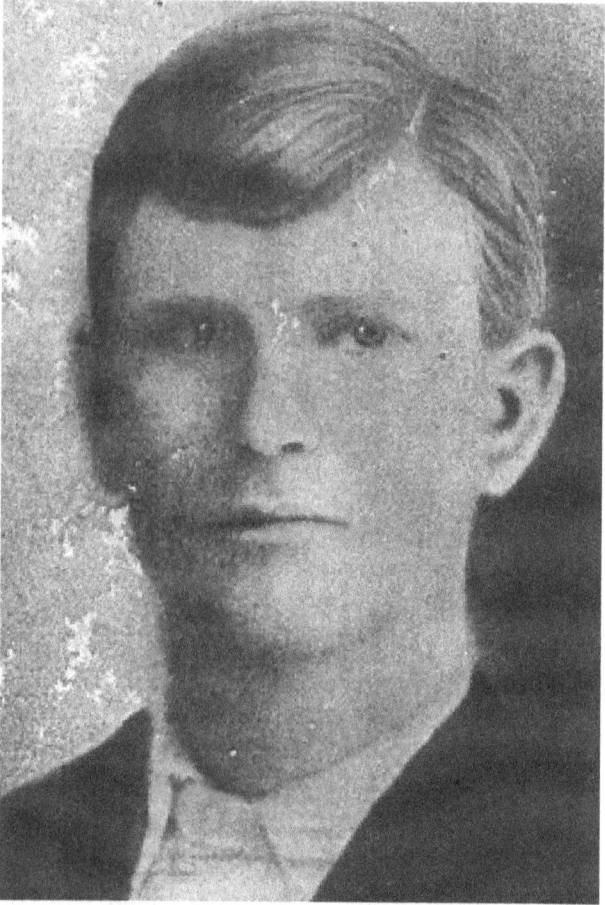

Dennis Peter O'Leary, Survivor

Chas Anderson of Fruto, California, vomited during the party and sought medical attention in Willows the next day. He also recovered and no further ill effects were reported about him. However, Cash Martin and Andy O'Leary were not so fortunate. Cash and Andy became progressively more ill as the days passed.

Frank was the first to die of botulism. During his last days, the *Colusa Sun-Herald* newspaper reported that Frank "suffered intensely" and was said to be "burned up with an awful thirst that could not be assuaged." The newspaper reported that he "passed away in terrible agony" in the hospital on Monday, September 20, 1919. Frank Carney died of cardiac failure nine days after drinking wine containing botulinum toxin.

Even at the time of Frank's death, Jack's condition was reported as "critical but the chances for his recovery are fair." After a brief hospitalization, Jack was taken to the home of his brother, Eli Triplett, in Maxwell, where he passed away on Tuesday, September 22, 1919. Andrew Jackson "Jack" Triplett died of cardiac failure eleven days after drinking wine containing botulinum toxin.

Sixteen days after the party, Cash Martin and Andy O'Leary were both hospitalized in Colusa. Dr. Frank L. Kelly from the California State Health Department, an expert on botulism, arrived from Berkeley to examine the last two men. After reviewing the clinical charts, Dr. Kelly said, "It was impossible to make a forecast. The men have chances of recovery if they can fight off the poison a little longer, they might come through all right and get entirely well."

Andrew "Andy" Jackson O'Leary, age thirty-three, was a native of Stonyford. He was the son of Mr. and Mrs. Jeremiah O'Leary. Andy had returned in June of 1919 from the Great War. He had fought for two years serving in the 144th Machine Gun Battalion and the 119th Machine Gun Battalion. He also fought bravely in the

Argonne Forest fight, which was the last major battle of the war.

Andy had politely partaken of the "well-meant hospitality" offered at the Triplet Ranch over the weekend. He worked all day in the hayfield with his brother on Monday. Toward evening, he complained that his throat "felt queer," but he often had throat troubles, so he thought little about his ailment. However, that night his throat felt numb. The next morning his brother took him to the physician in the nearby town of Willows. The physician examined Andy and sent him home; his condition continued to worsen. When Andy found out about the illnesses of Frank, Jack, and Cash, he realized the homebrewed wine was to blame.

Andy's family took him to the hospital in Colusa, where they remained by his side night and day. He was the "idol of his family, loved by innumerable friends." Dr. Rathbun and Dr. Poage quickly diagnosed Andy as poisoned by "botulinis" [sic], which they called a "rare, strange, and baffling malady." Andy had consumed very little of the poison wine, but his constitution was thought to be "shattered by his hard experiences in the Great War." The *Colusa Sun-Herald* newspaper reported Andy's plight:

> "The young man fought with all his energy to throw off the grip of the toxine [sic]. As stoically as a soldier stricken on the battlefield, he suffered without complaint. But a time came when, as he grew weaker, he seemed to know that the struggle was in vain. Several times during the night before the end, he told

his brother that he would not live.
Words of cheer at first had given
him fresh hope, but at last they
could not drive away the knowledge
of the approaching end."

On the following morning, while
Andy's worn-out brother-who had been
standing vigil-was sleeping, a
faithful nephew left Andy for a
moment to go fetch some ice. He
seemed just the same as he had been
for hours. Upon returning to the
sickroom only a moment later, the
nephew found Andy passing away.

This is the typical ending of those
stricken with botulinus poisoning.
Paralysis creeps nearer and nearer to
the vital nerve centers until life is
suddenly snuffed out."

Andrew "Andy" Jackson O'Leary died suddenly on October 1, 1919, after battling botulism for eighteen days.

Cash Martin was the final fatality of the outbreak, but he left his written musings behind. He had come from Ohio and worked for the railroad. He also worked as a land surveyor and auctioneer. He had fought in the Spanish-American War, serving in the Philippines. There it was reported "a savage islander in a vanguard skirmish struck him in the face with a bolo leaving a scar that would go with him to the tomb." Cash was more writer than farmer, living a simple and joyful life in the foothills of Stonyford, California.

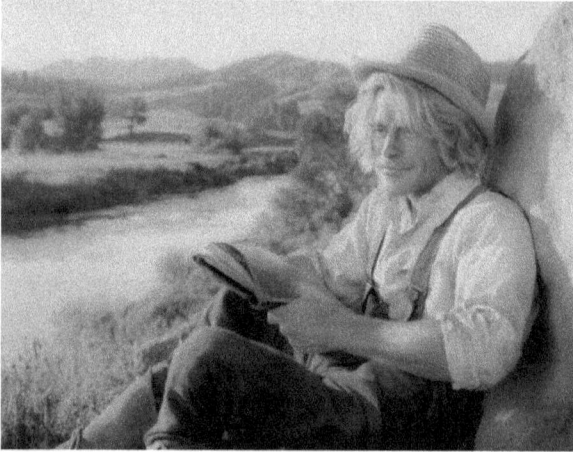

Cash Martin
Image generated using MidJourney AI

Once Cash was settled in California, he worked
as a correspondent for the local newspapers in the
towns of Willows and Colusa. His columns were
known for reciting "with humor and pathos the
happiness and tribulations of mountain folk." The
Colusa Daily Sun newspaper extolled the virtues
and talents of Cash Martin:

> "Martin was somewhat of a literary
> genius and did considerable writing
> for several of the papers in his
> section. He was a lover of nature, a
> dreamer, and a man of considerable
> originality in thought; and from his
> mountain home at Stonyford, where he
> was a hill farmer, he sent out his
> thoughts to the people in the
> valleys, and what he wrote was ever
> worth perusal."

After ten days of botulinum toxin ravaging his body, Cash was confined to his hospital bed and unable to speak; he wrote a farewell column to his readers on September 25. It seemed like an explanation for what he hoped would be a temporary absence from the newspaper. At this point, Cash had not been told about the death of his friends.

HIS FAREWELL.

Probably the last—may not be; but, anyway, here I am once more.

You people of the mountains, plains and everywhere, who read this, may God bless you. I have always loved my readers, else should not have written.

I am over at the Busch hospital in Calousa and never received better treatment in my life, or more warm-hearted friends.

Oh, how my heart hones and my sense of hearing would like to hear the sun-kissed wild waters of old Stony as she sings sweet lullabys for all who pass near her.

People of Stonyford, I love you all. Goodbye—for a time.

Cash Martin.

Cash lingered for another week in the hospital after writing the brief farewell column. On October 1, his physician reported that Cash was somewhat improved. On October 3, he reported that Cash "had a chance of recovering." Cassius Edwin Martin, age fifty-three, died on October 4, 1919, after a twenty-day battle with botulism. He passed away at the hour the funeral for his friend Andy was taking place in Stonyford. Cash was buried in the Colusa cemetery, fifty miles from his beloved Stony Creek.

His wife, Jeanie, became a forty-three-year-old widow that day. He also left behind his son, Miles, who had graduated from eighth grade the previous spring. His daughter, Goldie, was only four years old. The *Colusa Daily Sun* newspaper indulged its readers with an entertaining story that Cash had written early in the illness while joking about their folly, not realizing it would turn deadly. Cash wrote:

> "Two Stonyford men the other day decided there was no law against placing some canned preserves - apricots, peaches and the like - in a bar'l, and no law against filling said bar'l with genuine old Stony Creek water. Furthermore, Uncle Sam could have no objections to the combination sitting a few days. Looking through the Declaration of Independence, the constitution of the realm, the book of statutes and the National Prohibition Weekly, they found no law against drinking from a bar'l.
>
> So far, so good.
>
> They drank. As they did so the gloom of life vanished. The manzanita turned to porphery [sic], the

chemisal [sic] to onyx, the liveoak
bush to frankincense. Roses bloomed
afresh, fountains sprayed perfume,
and untold wealth was theirs. That
stuff about Bolsheviks,
reactionaries, influenza and wars
and horrors slunk away, and they
lived once more in the glorious days
of 1889.

But finally the bar'l went dry.
Sobering up set in. It set in like a
third battle of the Marne. The world
came back to reality. A Calousa
doctor was called. Their throats
were paralyzed; their brows were
fevered. They were, in brief,
strictly sick. It is believed they
will recover, but for a time it was
not altogether certain."

The tale didn't end the way Cash Martin
predicted in the early stages of his illness.

This homebrew outbreak in September of
1919 occurred on the heels of a high-profile
botulism outbreak the previous month in August
in Canton, Ohio. Awareness and documentation
regarding botulism was on the rise in the medical
literature. The medical community was quickly
becoming proficient at diagnosing botulism due
to the quality of documentation generated by
each botulism outbreak.

Dr. Rathbun, the local physician, called in a
botulism expert from Berkeley, Dr. Frank Kelly,
who was a colleague of the eminent Dr. J.C.
Geiger, a leading botulism scientist who worked
for the U.S. Public Health Department.
Developing expertise in diagnosing botulism was

possible because Dr. E.C. Dickson of Stanford University (the location of an earlier outbreak in 1913) had published substantial information about botulism in 1918.

Dr. Kelly traveled over one hundred miles from Berkeley to Colusa and examined the two patients still alive, gathering background on those who had passed away and who had recovered. He published a summary in the California State Health Board bulletin in October of 1919. It is interesting to note that this botulism outbreak did not make the national news and was not published in a national medical journal as the other outbreaks were. This could have been because illegal alcohol was involved during Prohibition.

The California bulletin reported that all six of the victims in the homebrew botulism outbreak displayed double vision and generalized muscle weakness. All of the men had sore throats and difficulties swallowing. Eventually, the four men hospitalized lost the ability to speak. At times, some showed rapid pulse and rapid respiration. Most had fevers; one man's fever was 102.6. Fever is atypical of botulism intoxication, but it is possible with a secondary infection.

Two of the four fatal cases were from cardiac failure due to botulism. Fatal botulism is most closely associated with respiratory collapse caused by a paralyzed diaphragm, but modern research shows that cardiac events are fairly common in fatal botulism cases. The heart is a muscle; botulinum toxin weakens the muscle and can disrupt the electrical system of the heart.

The damage to the cardiac function was established by early botulinum toxin researchers in France in 1897. Almost one hundred years later, a medical publication from the Center for Disease Control in 1987 reflected that half of the botulism deaths in their study were the result of delayed cardiac-related fatalities, not the initial respiratory challenges.

Dr. Kelly made an astute observation seldom mentioned in medical literature reflecting the waxing and waning of symptoms, noting, "Reflexes varied at times, being ceased at one time and diminished at others." An important atypical symptom of botulism noted was left-sided hemiplegia in two of the fatal cases. Modern medicine now commonly characterizes botulism as presenting as "symmetrical descending paralysis," but there are many reports in the early medical literature about paralysis occurring only on one side of the body. The early medical literature was focused on capturing every diagnostic detail of patients' cases, so physicians would learn to recognize botulism quickly.

Botulism is an extraordinary disease that stuns people. In the course of life, people fall ill occasionally for short periods of time with a variety of afflictions, most minor. They rest, they recover, and they resume their normal lives. When people are poisoned by botulinum toxin, such as these gentlemen were in 1919, they assume that they have some ordinary, run-of-the-mill illness or routine food poisoning.

While botulism is often thought of as swift and severe, history provides examples that mild botulism and delayed onset of botulism are equally as deadly as the swift variety.

TAKEAWAYS from
THE HOMEBREW OUTBREAK

Botulism can cause death in a matter of days or a matter of weeks.

Botulism symptoms unfold at a different pace for each patient and can also present with different severities for each patient. Even when all cases experience fatal outcomes, the progression varies greatly.

Botulism patients often underestimate their condition's severity; sudden decline and death can surprise both patient and physician.

Botulism symptoms wax and wane, which gives hope for recovery, only to suddenly result in a fatal outcome.

Vomiting the offending food after consumption can prove life-saving.

Cardiac-related deaths in botulism are common.

CHAPTER 7

Four Doctors, Four Different Diagnoses
THE DETROIT, MICHIGAN
OUTBREAK of 1919

On Saturday, October 18, 1919, the prominent Sales family of Detroit hosted a dinner party for six of their close friends at their home near the shores of Lake St. Clair in Grosse Pointe, Michigan.

This small gathering would end in tragedy and be featured nationally in the newspapers, with the world's biggest media conglomerate, the Hearst Corporation, publishing a grim headline about the botulism poisoning and deaths that resulted. "Death Came Unbidden to Mrs. Sales' Dinner Party" warned readers about an odorless, tasteless killer in canned food. The full-page story, illustrated with a wealthy couple being served olives by a skeleton in a maid's uniform, appeared in newspapers nationwide. Seven people at the Sales' party ate Curtis brand ripe black olives and were stricken with botulism; five of them died within one week and two recovered.

Public interest around the outbreak was high; it seemed unthinkable that such tragedy could befall a family of such good fortune. Prior to the botulism outbreak, the Sales family led idyllic lives in a world wrought with disease and war. Murray W. Sales, the father, was a prominent industrialist in Detroit, Michigan, who had worked his way into the wholesale plumbing business. Their home, the site of the dinner, was an 11,181-square-foot mansion designed by architect Louis Kamper commissioned by Murray in 1917. Mansions of this stature had names, and this one was known as "Edgeroad."

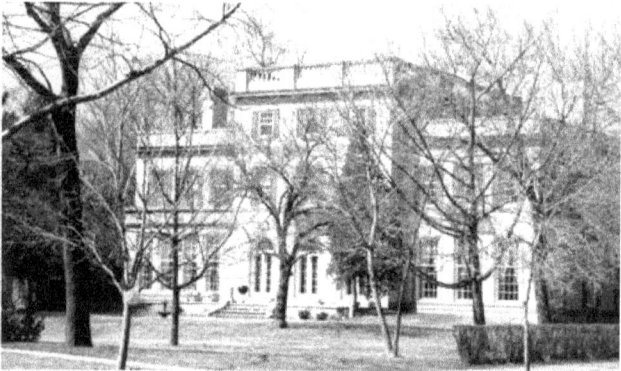

Edgeroad: family home of the Sales family

As a teen, Murray had started as an office boy for the dry goods firm Allan Sheldon & Company; eventually he took the job of representative for the Detroit Copper and Brass Rolling Company. He then became the co-founder of the Murray W. Sales Company, a wholesale plumbing firm. Murray Sales also served on the board of directors of several companies: Michigan Bell Telephone Company, Manufacturers' National Bank, Michigan Consolidated Gas Company, National Steel Corporation, and Detroit Steel Products Company.

On Christmas Day of 1892, Murray married Jessie Carter, daughter of the president of Detroit & Cleveland Navigation Company. She was described in the newspapers as a "socialite belle." Murray and Jessie lost their first-born child as an infant, then raised four more children. Jessie held prestigious society positions in The Neighborhood Club. An active socialite, she maintained a constant presence at tea parties and garden club events while servants helped her maintain the household at the mansion.

At the time of the botulism outbreak, the eldest son, Carter Sales, was twenty-five years old. He had miraculously returned home safely from the Great War just one year prior and had earned a degree at the University of Michigan. Frances Sales, age twenty-three and their only daughter, was considered a prominent young "society woman" within the musical and social circles of Detroit. Murray Sales, Jr., age sixteen, was Princeton University bound. Leonard Sales, the youngest, was only twelve years old.

The dinner party would see the Sales family hosting six socially prominent leaders from Detroit: the Newberrys (John and Edith), the Lewises (Ingersoll and Bertha), and the Curries (Cameron and Harriette). Harriette Currie was the sister of Ingersoll Lewis. The wives–Jessie Sales, Edith Newberry, Harriette Currie, and Bertha Lewis–socialized together frequently and were featured regularly in the society pages of the Detroit newspapers.

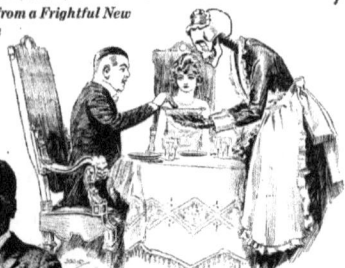

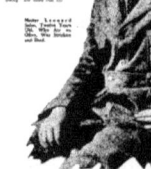

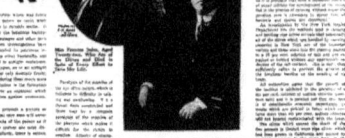

The meal on October 18th required not only the family's usual maid, Miss Julia Manes, but additional help. Barbara Cassell was hired as an additional household helper for the dinner.

The menu included a delicacy: canned ripe black olives from California. The same black olives were also served on the following Sunday on Frances' twenty-third birthday.

The Fatal Cases

Barbara Cassell, the additional maid, showed signs of illness on Sunday; she was reported to have "a slight difficulty of vision, pain in the head, and nervousness." By noon, she had difficulty swallowing. Her family physician examined her at 3:00 PM, but found no objective symptoms of disease. By 7:00 PM Sunday evening, Barbara's symptoms intensified; she vomited and had abdominal pain, and had diarrhea. Her physician described her as "hysterical," but thought it was because of a domestic misunderstanding that had occurred just a few hours earlier. Monday she continued to decline. By 10:00 PM Monday night, Barbara Helen Cassell, age thirty-two, collapsed and died, just forty-eight hours after consuming olives containing botulinum toxin. Even for botulism, this is a steep death curve. The others from the dinner party had no knowledge of her illness or passing.

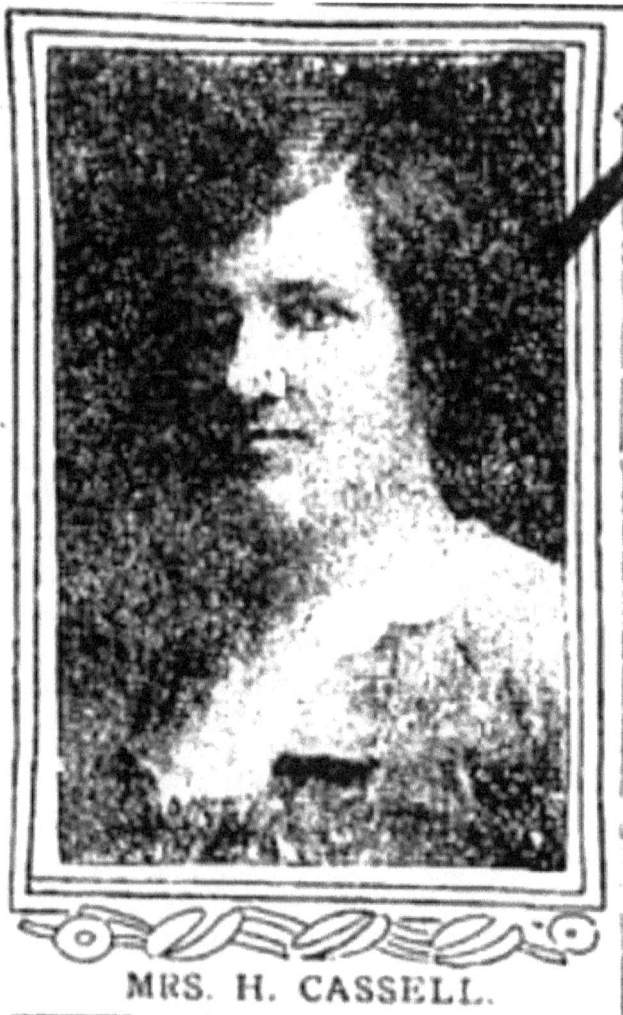

MRS. H. CASSELL.

Barbara Helen Cassell

Alexander "Ingersoll" Lewis was a dear friend of Murray Sales. One of thirteen children, a Yale University graduate, and a son of the former Mayor of Detroit, Ingersoll was a capitalist and a prominent town father. He held various business positions in the Newland Hat Company, the Liberty Motor Car Company, and the Morris Plan Bank.

Ingersoll began to feel ill while playing golf on Sunday. He reported vision difficulties during the game. Upon returning home, Ingersoll said he had never felt more tired in his life. On Monday, he experienced double vision and had difficulty articulating his words. On Tuesday, he had difficulty swallowing. He had ptosis in his right eyelid and a "lazy eye" in the right eye. His pupils were dilated and reacted slowly to light. The right side of Ingersoll's face was paralyzed. On Wednesday, dyspnea set in, and he was having trouble breathing, feeling as if he could not get enough air. Along with that, he had laryngospasm that created a choking sensation that made breathing and speaking nearly impossible.

On Thursday, Alexander Ingersoll Lewis, age forty-five, died due to "cerebral thrombosis and softening" according to his family physician, who would find no reasonable explanation for this death. His physicians commented that Ingersoll "was in excellent health, and presented no cardiovascular disease or syphilis." He left behind his wife, Bertha Antoinette, and three children, Elizabeth, age seventeen, and twins Alexander and Annette, age twelve.

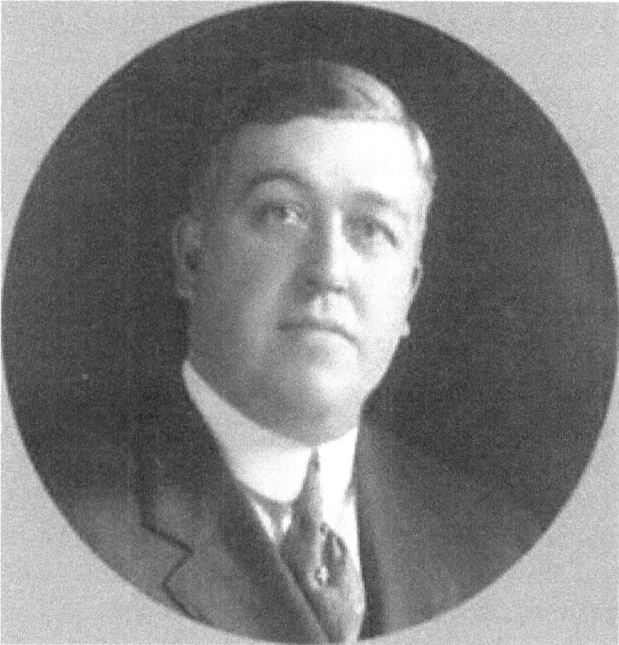

Alexander Ingersoll Lewis

Jessie Sales and her two children were also violently ill that week with what presented as food poisoning. Leonard had eaten olives Sunday, Monday, and Tuesday. On Wednesday, he vomited and then felt more comfortable. By Wednesday night, he had a dimness of vision and double vision. He had traveled by automobile that day and had trouble navigating his way from the driveway back into the mansion. Leonard's condition deteriorated Wednesday evening. He vomited again at 7:00 PM. He had a severe convulsion lasting for about one minute around 8:30 PM. He vomited once more after the convulsion. After that, he could not swallow or speak and had marked muscle weakness. Leonard Adam Sales, age twelve, failed quickly and died at 3:00 AM Thursday morning, just twelve hours after his first symptom appeared. His death reflected the fact that botulinum toxin can have a delayed onset of a few days and then manifest rapidly into a death spiral in less than a day.

Julia Manes, the maid, age forty-three, also ate olives on Sunday, Monday, and Tuesday. On Wednesday, she vomited and experienced abdominal pain. Julia felt that eating olives relieved her nausea, so she kept eating them. She also developed dimness of vision, double vision, and difficulty swallowing. These symptoms lasted for twenty-four hours and during that time, the symptoms would "clear up almost completely." This waxing and waning of symptoms is quite common in botulism; it gives the patient false hope of recovery while the illness progresses toward a fatal outcome.

On Thursday morning, Julia vomited blood. By noon, she had lost the ability to swallow and had ptosis of the left eyelid. Nystagmus, uncontrolled rapid eye movements, was present. As the afternoon passed, she became very weak and had difficulty breathing. For Julia to survive, it was "necessary to use all the accessory muscles of respiration." By evening, Julia had fallen into a semi-coma. Her pulse was "rapid, weak, and irregular." She lingered another day before dying at 10:30 PM on Friday night in Harper Hospital. Cause of death was listed as cardiac and respiratory paralysis.

Frances Sales, who celebrated her twenty-third birthday that Sunday, ate a total of two olives over the period of Sunday and Monday. On Wednesday, she noticed coryza (an inflammation of the respiratory track), sore throat, blurry vision, and double vision. However, Frances told others that she did not feel sick. On Thursday, she felt weak. At noon, she started to eat soup, but could not swallow it. Immediately, she felt nauseated and vomited once. Because of her dimness of vision and weakness, she had to be assisted to bed. The ptosis of both eyelids was so severe that Frances had to throw back her head to see through the slits of her eyelids There was no paralysis of the face or tongue. A thick layer of mucus had accumulated in the throat that she could neither expel nor swallow. Her mental state was clear. Frances rested well Thursday evening.

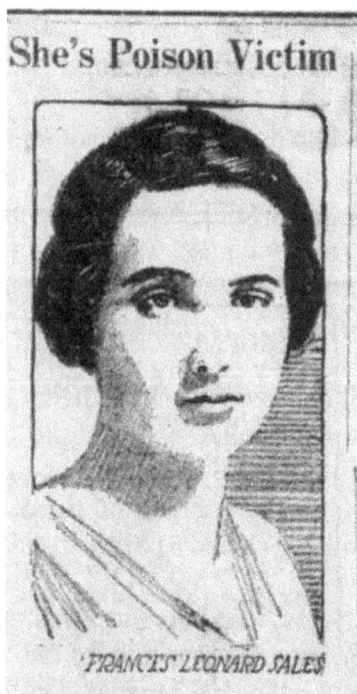

She's Poison Victim

FRANCES LEONARD SALES

Frances Sales

On Friday morning, Frances was weaker, but the ptosis was less severe, and she was comfortable all morning. However, by noon, she complained that she was "smothering." Her respiration became "wholly thoracic and labored with the accessory respiratory muscles in play." The mucus became more annoying. With the respiration difficulties, Frances became more anxious and restless.

On Saturday, Frances was "clear mentally, but drowsy and almost too weak to move." Her speech had been fairly clear up to this point, but became very indistinct. The tongue was swollen and could not be protruded. Her hands felt numb, so she rubbed them to restore circulation.

The botulism antitoxin serum developed by Professor Robert Graham at the University of Illinois was rushed by special messenger from Champaign, Illinois, to Detroit, Michigan, and administered to Frances on Saturday. It had no effect. The antitoxin was still in the experimental stage in 1919. Within a few years, it was determined the 1919 version of Dr. Graham's botulism antitoxin was specific to a botulinum toxin type B only (not type A) and therefore ineffective on the strain of botulism Frances had.

Her physician reported that "she suddenly became cloudy mentally and pulse rose to 160." Shortly thereafter, Frances became comatose for three hours, during which time she partially aroused for brief times. Frances Sales died of respiration paralysis six days after she had eaten the leftover olives.

A double funeral was held for the children on Monday morning at the Sales family home. Though their mother, Jessie, was severely ill, she was able to attend her children's funerals.

The Survivors

Jessie Sales, age forty-eight, ate a small portion of one olive at the dinner party on Saturday and a whole olive the next day. On Tuesday, she had a haziness of vision and double vision. On Wednesday, she had difficulty swallowing solid food and moderate ptosis of the right eyelid. On Saturday, the botulism antitoxin was also administered to Jessie, but it made no impact on her condition. The newspapers described her as "recovered very slowly from nervous and muscular debility."

Bertha Lewis, age forty-three, ate a small portion of one olive on Saturday. She developed symptoms of poisoning on Tuesday. She had "slightly disturbed vision, mild ptosis, obstinate constipation, and difficulty swallowing solid food." Bertha's symptoms were not severe, and she recovered in a few days.

Harriette Currie felt no ill effects from the meal.

Edith Newberry had heeded a casual warning about the olives from Cameron Currie, the guest seated next to her. He remarked to Edith, "this olive seems to be a trifle overripe." The newspaper reported that Jessie made a "light retort to the criticism of her guest, but she ate an olive and Saturday showed some symptoms of poisoning."

Aside from Cameron Currie and Ingersoll Lewis, the other men at the dinner party did not eat any olives.

The Misdiagnoses

Murray Sales told the newspapers that his son's death was diagnosed as ptomaine poisoning by the family physician. When the relatives of Barbara Cassell read about Leonard's death in the newspapers, they called Murray. Barbara's physician had been puzzled and suggested poisoning earlier, but his suspicions were dismissed at the time.

The cause of death for the first two victims, Barbara Cassel and Ingersoll Lewis, remained inconclusive until the cases were discussed by all four physicians: Dr. E.R. Witwer, Dr. J.A. Belanger, the family physician for the Sales family), and the father-son duo Dr. A.F. Jennings and his son, Dr. C.G. Jennings. They met on Friday and discussed the unusual circumstances of the deaths of the five patients that week, as well as the symptoms of the others stricken after the meal at Edgeroad. Behind closed doors, they suspected botulism, but they decided to contact the laboratories at the University of Michigan to reach a definitive diagnosis.

A toxicity test was performed on guinea pigs on Friday afternoon by order of the health commissioner Dr. V.C. Vaughan. Dr. Herbert Emmerson at the University of Michigan medical school and his assistant, George Collins, conducted the test. Four guinea pigs were each given seven drops of black olive juice by means of a stomach pump; all four guinea pigs displayed botulism symptoms and died within fourteen hours. Other pigs were given a larger dose of botulinum toxin-laced olive juice and died in a shorter time. Dr.

Emmerson continued to experiment in an effort to find the smallest dose that would be fatal to guinea pigs. These laboratory tests confirmed the physicians' theory; the cause of deaths from the dinner at the Edgeroad mansion was botulinum toxin.

By the Monday following the five deaths from the Sales' dinner party, health officials in Detroit had seized seven-thousand jars of olives from local retail store shelves. The packing liquid in one of those jars of olives proved fatal in the other guinea pig experiments; the pigs died of botulism within thirty minutes of being injected. Toxicity tests involved oral administration, but injection yielded faster results. By early December of 1919, over twenty-thousand cases of olives in Michigan alone were impounded by the state.

The Press

A month after the deaths, the "Detroit Outbreak" became the center of a national botulism awareness campaign published across the U.S. in newspapers owned by the Hearst Corporation. The storyline explained this strange newly identified public health threat–odorless and tasteless–residing in canned food. These botulism scares occurred around the same time as the Spanish Flu, so the newspapers published stories with great detail explaining how an illness from botulinum toxin was different from a viral infection. The Hearst story reflected the role of the press in the national communication effort around educating and warning the public about botulism:

"What killed them? They were victims of a strange new food poison newly discovered and called botulism – a poison produced by the recently identified bacillius botulinus.

They did not swallow germs which began to breed and poison them. The deadly poison was already all there on those olives – a tasteless, odorless, invisible but frightfully potent poison. That is one of the strange things about this poison – the microbe in the food makes the poison and deposits it in the food. It is not the microbe that hurts you; it is the poison it has put in the food before you eat it.

It is a strange uncanny germ. It cannot live in the air; it does not thrive or give off the poison in the warmth of the body. The bacillius botulinus may be eaten without danger. The germ lives and breeds and creates its poison in the sealed can or jar where there is no air, no oxygen.

Science knows no cure for this poison. There is no way that the housewife nor the guest can tell whether the poison is in the food. But there are some things which everybody ought to know and to do to guard against this new food poison which struck with deadly effect, Mrs. Sales' dinner party.

Totally different in symptoms and far more fatal in character than "ptomaine poisoning," which is of frequent occurrence, this serious and

seldom encountered poisoning is one
of which the public has little, if
any, knowledge either as to the
causes or symptoms or means of
prevention. Cases may be much more
common than the records show. Few
doctors know this disease and many
cases may have occurred which were
not recognized.

Within twenty-four hours the victims
began to be stricken. Medical
specialists diagnosed the illness
correctly, but they were helpless -
there was nothing they could do."

As applicable today as it was in 1919, "Cases may be much more common than the records show. Few doctors know this disease and many cases may have occurred which were not recognized." This quote in the Hearst newspaper story echoes Dr. Wilbur's observation from the 1913 outbreak at Stanford: "The isolated case is the one that is most apt to lead to confusion and misdiagnosis."

During the course of one week, Murray Sales watched his family suffer from botulism, buried his best friend, and realized the gathering at his home had caused the deaths of two maids who served the family. By the end of the week, Murray stood by helplessly as his only daughter, his youngest son, and his beloved wife struggled to breathe while botulism paralyzed the nerves of their diaphragm muscles. It was a slow and merciless strangulation. His son died first. Then his ill daughter showed signs of improvement, but then perished next. Only his wife, Jessie, survived the ordeal.

Three months after the children's deaths and on the heels of the Bronx botulism outbreak, the newspaper reported the status of Murray Sales:

"He was prepared to spend much time, energy, and money to prevent further loss of life from this cause. Reports of five deaths in New York from botulinus poisoning last week hastened this decision Mr. Sales explained. He said he has felt for some time that it is a duty he owes humanity."

Murray and Jessie Sales coped with the tragedy and death of their children by helping others through philanthropy and community service; prior to losing Leonard and Frances to botulism in 1919, they had also lost their firstborn child at just thirteen days old in 1902. Motivated by these losses, Jessie co-founded The Cottage Hospital in Grosse Pointe with her husband Murray; their family physician Dr. Alpheus F. Jennings; and other local philanthropists. Jessie served as President of The Cottage Hospital. Murray and Jessie sponsored the children's wing in honor of their three deceased children. Jessie also served in leadership for The Neighborhood Club, which was "a mecca for east side children seeking happiness." Over one thousand children paid the dues of twenty-five cents per year. The club raised money to construct a building for use by thirty different youth groups including, Boy Scouts, Gardeners' club, Chauffeurs' Club, Blue Birds, V.V.V. Girls, Camp Fire Girls, Dramatic Club, and basketball leagues.

Murray Sales gave repeated interviews to the press to keep the public apprised of his commitment to resolve the public health threat from botulinum toxin. The local newspaper reported:

> "While the dual blow seemed one from which it would be almost impossible to recover, Mr. Sales rallied his forces to meet courageously the condition and, moreover, since that time has put forth untiring effort before Congress and elsewhere in order to eliminate the possibility of the deadly botulismus [sic] germ invading canned products in the future."

Two years after the tragedy in Detroit in 1919, another deadly botulism outbreak from canned spinach in Grand Rapids, Michigan, prompted these comments from Murray Sales:

> "My efforts, I believe, soon will have tangible results. There is pending in Congress a bill designed to place under federal supervision all packing houses and factories in which such foods may convey poison are prepared. This would take the matter out of the hands of those states which now exercise supervision. The bill was prepared in cooperation with the department of justice in Washington and is now, I understand, in conference.
>
> It is not because I expect ever again to be afflicted personally in that

way, but for the sake of humanity and
for others, I am determined to do all
in my power to lessen the fatalities
caused by those who think less of
human life than of profits."

Four years after the Edgeroad tragedy, in 1923, the society pages reported that Murray and Jessie resumed taking their summers at the beach cottage on St. Louis Row in Pointe Aux Barques. Life would not be the same, but it would go on. The advocacy work around food safety was a constant crusade in Murray's life. The newspapers reported his progress:

"Mr. Sales is informed that certain
persons have gone so far as to seek
to prevent publicity of the official
warnings to consumers. 'This is
terrible,' he exclaimed, 'to think of
caring more for dollars and cents
than for humanity.

This poison is the most deadly one
and people should be warned again and
again to exercise the greatest care
in buying and preparing canned foods.
Newspapers must do their part in the
campaign of warning and education,
and papers which resist pressure put
upon them by those interested more in
profits than the welfare of humanity
are to be highly commended.

The olive firm which was responsible
for the deaths a year or so ago now
is in financial difficulties."

After the botulism tragedy in their home, the future held even more loss for Murray Sales. His middle son, Murray Jr., died in 1926 at age twenty-three while returning from a dance. His automobile struck a utility pole. An investigation later revealed a warning flasher had been removed for repairs earlier that afternoon. His wife Jessie died in 1943, one week after their 50th wedding anniversary. The sole surviving son, Carter, died of a heart attack in 1944 at age fifty while exercising at a gymnasium. In 1944, Murray was seventy-nine years old and all of his immediate family members were gone. He spent his remaining time until his death at eighty-five contributing to his community through friendship and projects to help children. The obituary for Murray Sales explained his philanthropy toward underprivileged children:

> "With his family gone, Mr. Sales found comfort in his declining years in the association of lifetime friends. For seventeen years, he joined James F. Holden in sponsoring the Detroit Christmas Party."

So much was taken from Murray Sales, yet he continued to find ways to give to others. He was the activist responsible for public policy around food safety laws that were informed by science from and The Botulism Commission. To some degree, even the food supply used by the Allied Forces in World War II benefited from the advocacy of Murray Sales; canned foods became vastly safer to eat. He channeled his pain into protecting others and improving the lives of children.

TAKEAWAYS from
THE DETROIT OUTBREAK

Individual cases of botulism are routinely misdiagnosed.

Paralysis is not always symmetrical.

Asymmetrical paralysis can result in one eyelid having ptosis and the other not being affected.

Victims who don't feel sick or look sick to others can unknowingly be in a death spiral.

Botulism victims underestimate the severity of their illness.

Botulism is often misdiagnosed when the individuals in a botulism outbreak are treated by different physicians.

Botulism outcomes range from mild to severe to fatal.

Recovery from botulism can take days or years.

Within a single outbreak, patients share some symptoms but often have differing symptoms.

Patients underestimate the seriousness of a botulism intoxication. Early in the illness, they often don't feel extremely sick, but can quickly succumb to a steep decline in health, which leads to death.

Seizures are a prelude to death. Seizures are evidence that botulinum toxin has spread to the brain.

A seriously ill patient can show a slight improvement for a few hours, then suddenly die.

CHAPTER 8

The Walking Dead
THE BRONX, NEW YORK
OUTBREAK of 1920

The Curtis Corporation's ripe black olives struck in January of 1920, killing nearly every member of the Delbene family within days of consumption. The family, immigrants from Noci in southern Italy, made their fortune as shoemakers in New York City after having immigrated to the United States in 1905. While most of the family lived in the Bronx, one of the brothers, Dominick, lived in Manhattan.

Dominick would sometimes celebrate his visits to his brother, Paul Delbene's family, by bringing glass jars of olives as a delicacy for the entire family. Such had been the case when Maria Delbene, Paul's wife and the mother of the household, became violently ill on the night of Friday, January 9, 1920.

Maria was particularly fond of olives. She was known for sneaking this treat while preparing meals. Maria alone partook of the coveted olives, then she was struck with stomach upset and vomiting at 10 PM Friday night. She spent the entire night crying, vomiting, and worrying.

A doctor arrived at the home at 8:00 AM and found Maria unable to swallow. Her vision was blurred. There was no pain in her abdomen and her throat looked normal. She experienced choking sensations and partial blindness. The doctor was called back to the house at 12:00 PM and found Maria dead.

Her husband Paul told the doctor that Maria had been treated for kidney issues for the past two years. Her death certificate listed the dimness of vision as "albuminuric retinitis" and listed the cause of death as "uremia and chronic nephritis." Maria Delbene, age thirty-three, died on Saturday, January 10, 1920, just fourteen hours after symptoms developed. Poisoning was not suspected as the cause of death.

As funeral preparations began, the Delbenes youngest son, Joseph, age seven, was sent away to be cared for at a friend's home. The others in the family remained home and mourned. A profound sadness enveloped the Bronx home at 2328 Hughes Avenue. During this time, the opened jar of olives Maria had eaten a few days earlier was found in a cabinet and used to prepare a salad on Tuesday evening. In addition, some of these same olives were placed on a plate as an appetizer. Another wave of illness descended upon the Delbene household following the funeral preparations. On Wednesday, January 14, three more family members suddenly became ill.

Maria and Paul Delbene's oldest son, Dominica, age sixteen, developed symptoms similar to his mother's. He was seized by a choking sensation, the inability to swallow, partial loss of vision, vomiting, and extreme weakness. He could not speak, but was able to communicate by writing. Dominica was unable to open his eyes due to ptosis of both eyelids. His pulse was 80, but very weak. The physician recorded these symptoms at 7:00 AM that day. Dominica was sent to Fordham Hospital at 10:00 AM by ambulance, but he died within thirty minutes of arrival. The hospital listed the diagnosis at admission as "paralysis of the throat, migraine, and hysteria." Dominica Delbene died Wednesday, January 14; he ate olives Tuesday night and was dead before noon on Wednesday.

It was upon completion of Dominica's autopsy that food poisoning was suspected. The physician remembered reading a recent article about olives causing a fatal botulism outbreak in Detroit, Michigan three months prior. This led to questioning the family's consumption of olives which led to the suspicion of botulism.

Within hours of Dominica's death on Wednesday morning, his father, Paul Delbene became ill. He had difficulty expectorating, dimness of vision, diplopia, prostration, weakness, difficulty swallowing, and glairy mucus in the throat. Despite his symptoms, he walked half a mile to the Fordham Hospital to seek treatment. His daughter Lena, age nine, accompanied him and was admitted to the hospital for observation. As the day unfolded, Paul developed ptosis, constipation, profuse perspiration, and aphonia (a loss of speech). Paul Delbene, age thirty-six, died on Friday morning, just two days after his symptoms presented. The father was the third Delbene to succumb to the poison.

Maria and Paul's middle son, Antonio Delbene, age thirteen, had become ill Wednesday evening. It was reported that he "became much alarmed when a sensation of choking developed in his throat." Despite two deaths in the family that week, or maybe because of it, Antonio walked to the Fordham Hospital at 4:45 AM on Thursday . Walking half a mile was likely a difficult task given how rapidly muscular paralysis can advance. The exertion may have increased the spread of toxin and muscle paralysis, which would have exacerbated his condition. He soon developed ptosis, dimness of vision, great weakness, prostration, aphonia, constipation, profuse perspiration, and glairy mucus in the throat. Antonio Delbene died on Friday, January 16.

That same Wednesday evening, Paul's younger brother, Angelo Delbene, age twenty-six, became ill. Angelo's first symptoms were dry throat, thick speech, difficult expectoration, and a choking sensation. Once admitted to the Fordham Hospital, he developed similar symptoms as his relatives, along with throat pain. Angelo Delbene died on Saturday, January 17.

The last to perish was Paul's oldest brother, Dominick, the Manhattan resident who originally purchased the olives. On Thursday, he felt "considerable apprehension" and experienced a "somewhat indefinite indisposition," as described by the physicians. He had already witnessed two of his family members mysteriously die that week, with three more hospitalized and struggling to survive. His first symptoms were "difficult expectoration and some dimness of vision." He also suffered a choking sensation.

Dominick also walked half a mile to the Fordham Hospital on Friday. Soon after his arrival, the death spiral began. His pupils were dilated and reacted sluggishly to light. He had muscle weakness, ptosis of both eyelids, difficulty speaking, constipation, profuse sweating, and a sense of chilliness. As his respiratory function began to fail, Dominick turned blue.

Meanwhile, public health officials scrambled on Friday to secure the antitoxin by airplane from Dr. Robert Graham at the University of Illinois, but mechanical difficulties and weather prevented its speedy delivery. The supply from Harvard University had been depleted, but they recommended the Bureau of Animal Industry in Washington, D.C. At last, Dr. Graham's antitoxin arrived and was immediately administered to Dominick; however, he died within hours.

The next week, laboratory tests showed Dr. Graham's antitoxin failed to protect guinea pigs that were fed the juice from the olives from the Delbene pantry. Later, it was discovered that this early antitoxin was only effective against botulinum toxin type B and the conclusion was drawn that the Delbenes died from botulinum toxin type A.

Dominick's mental status was described as "somewhat irrational" an hour before his death. Dominick Delbene, age forty-five, died on Saturday, January 17.

Similarities of the Fatal Cases

There were no survivors among those adults who ate the olives. The time to death was rapid, indicating they consumed several magnitudes of a lethal dose of botulinum toxin. All six of the fatal cases shared the following symptoms: ptosis of the eyelids, dimness of vision, muscle weakness, difficulty of speech, loss of voice, choking sensation, and constipation. Four out of five also experienced cyanosis from respiratory failure; that is, their skin took on a bluish tint from a lack of oxygen to the tissues.

Laboratory tests later determined the canned ripe olives found at the Delbene home were the source of the deadly botulinum toxin. Newspapers chronicled daily the saga of the botulism outbreak that ravaged the Delbene family. Only two of the children, Lena, age nine, and Joseph, age seven, survived the ordeal. Lena showed mild symptoms of botulism. She received two injections of the antitoxin, which was ultimately secured from Washington, D.C. Afterwards, she had a convulsion and developed a rash. Since Joseph had been with family friends and not in the household when the tainted olives were served, the decision was made to not administer the antitoxin to him.

It came to light that the olives sold to Dominick Delbene had been rejected as "not of good quality" by the New York distributor and were later resold by the California manufacturer. Thirty cases, or 720 jars of olives, had been sold in New York City. Soon after the Delbene tragedy, the press initiated a public awareness campaign about the dangers of canned ripe olives. News of this botulism outbreak that killed six people in the Bronx reached Murray Sales in Detroit and inspired him to continue his lobbying efforts for improved food safety laws.

TAKEAWAYS from
THE BRONX OUTBREAK

Misdiagnosis of individual botulism cases is common.

The cause of the first death was misdiagnosed despite showing neurological symptoms consistent with botulism.

Botulism presents a distinct set of neurological symptoms that can easily be misdiagnosed when the treating physician lacks direct experience with botulism.

There is variability in the symptoms even within the same botulism outbreak.

The tragedies developed the sense of urgency among public officials. Olives had caused multiple deaths in Ohio, Detroit, and New York City in six months. The entire canning industry was under pressure to assure a safe food supply.

Botulism patients often underestimate their condition's severity; sudden decline and death can surprise both patient and physician.

Complete respiratory collapse from botulism can happen with little to no warning, resulting in death within minutes.

CHAPTER 9

Corporate Greed = Deaths
THE MEMPHIS, TENNESSEE
OUTBREAK of 1920

The embroidery club of Memphis, Tennessee, met every Thursday with gatherings taking place at the homes of the members. Hosting responsibilities shifting among them. Responsibility for the luncheon on the February 5th, 1920 meeting fell to the club's newest member, Frances "Myrtle" Vunkannon.

The inclusion of Curtis brand canned ripe olives to the menu would result in the deaths of seven, including the hostess. Club members Elizabeth Jane Hammond, Robbie Crofford, Eugenia Ivy, and Myrtle Vunkannon, as well as two of their husbands and a child, would die as the result of the irresponsibility of the Curtis corporation.

Concerns over the influenza pandemic caused most of the members of the club to decline Myrtle's invitation; the decisions of Mrs. Frank Kerns, Mrs. Aubrey Olds, Mrs. Forrest Proctor, and Mrs. Cheairs Wilcox to not attend the embroidery club meeting undoubtedly saved their lives. Myrtle served ham sandwiches and a salad at her luncheon, prepared using Curtis brand olives purchased as a delicacy from Watson's Salvage store in Memphis. Disappointed by the low attendance, but not one to waste good food, Myrtle encouraged the two ladies who did show up to call their families and invite them over to eat the food.

Eugenia Ivy's young son, Currie, was recruited to share in the bounty of black olive sandwiches that Myrtle had so thoughtfully prepared. He bit into an olive, but was offended by the odor of the fruit. In the typical fashion of a nine-year-old, he replied, "Mother, that's nasty. I'm not going to eat any of them." He then "made a wry face and threw his olive away."

Eugenia's husband, Uzell Ivy, came by the Vunkannon home at 6:00 PM to take his wife home, but was persuaded by Max Vunkannon, his brother-in-law, to stay for supper. Max remarked that the olives were delicious. Max and Uzell "ate freely of the olives, laughingly remarking that the ladies had left such a large quantity of the delicious relish."

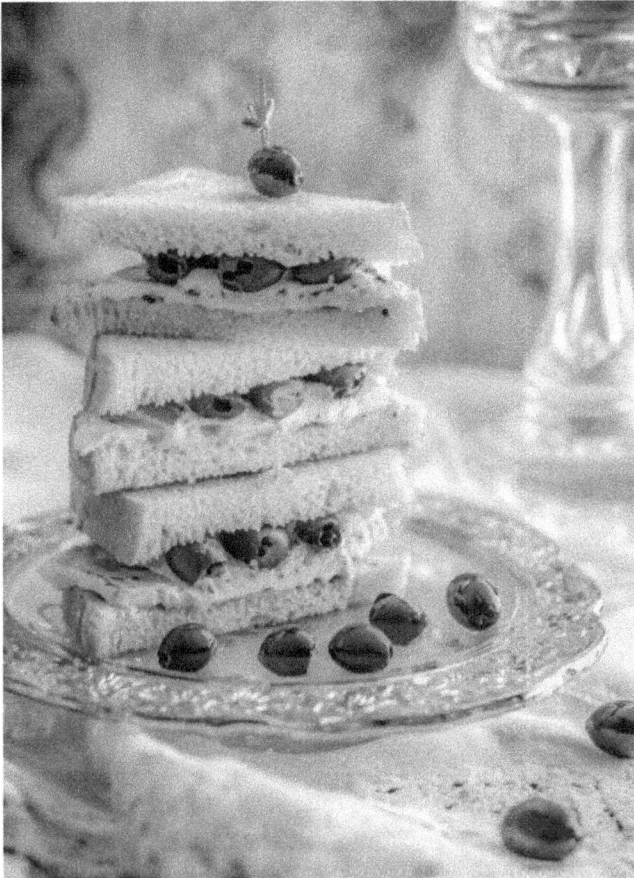

The first to die after the Thursday luncheon was Elizabeth Jane (Hardy) Hammond, the wife of Atlanta architect Horace B. Hammond. Elizabeth ate olives on Thursday afternoon and was dead the next day. Dr. A.R. McMahon reported Elizabeth was only sick for four hours prior to her death. She exhibited the signs of poisoning, but did not show the signs of ptomaine poisoning as there was no nausea or abdomen pain. He noted her symptoms were "paralysis of the nerves and muscles of the throat and the eyes and other indications that the brain cells were affected by the poison." The condition of the pupils led him to believe there was an active poison in her system. Dr. McMahon did not know the cause of death but speculated it might have been heart disease with goiter as a contributing factor. Elizabeth Jane (Hardy) Hammond, age forty-three, died at 8:30 AM on Friday and was buried in Evansville, Indiana.

Robbie Crofford complained of feeling dizzy Friday morning, but when she heard about the death of her friend Elizabeth, she came to Elizabeth's house to make preparations. Robbie was with friends at the Spencer Funeral Parlor at 7:00 PM Friday night when she was stricken with illness. Robbie (Cothran) Crofford, age twenty-nine, died at 6:10 AM Saturday morning. She was buried in Covington, Tennessee. She left behind her husband Herbert Sr. and one child, Herbert, Jr., age four.

After the illnesses of others at the Thursday gathering, authorities began to suspect olives as a source of poisoning. When Myrtle arose Friday morning, she was "almost blind," but she cooked breakfast anyway. She didn't feel well at all, but still completed her morning chores. At 3:00 PM that afternoon her brother, Uzell Ivy, was brought from work at the Belmont Candy Company to his sister's home and put to bed. He said he was "seeing two people for every one he looked at." He was cold and kept gasping for air.

Myrtle had grown worse as the day wore on, and her husband Max was summoned from his work to come home. When Max arrived, he dropped down into his chair and gasped for breath.

He did not speak to Myrtle or ask of her condition. When Myrtle realized her husband's condition, she exclaimed, "I'm going to die, brother's going to die, and Max is going to die."

Shortly thereafter, friends called Dr. Polk, who ordered Myrtle, Max, and Uzell to be transported to the hospital. While there, Myrtle joked that people would accuse her of drinking wood alcohol because she was seeing double.

Myrtle lost her voice to throat paralysis. In a gesture of love and to prepare her sister Minnie for the inevitable, Myrtle removed a ruby necklace from her neck and handed it to her sister. Myrtle silently mouthed the words "for baby, she's yours." Sensing her own oncoming death, Myrtle's final wishes were for Minnie to raise Myrtle's two-year-old daughter Maxine.

In the grips of botulism, victims sometimes have the mental clarity to understand what is happening and accept their approaching death. Frances "Myrtle" Vunkannon, age thirty-four, lost consciousness toward the end before dying at 5:55 AM Saturday. When the young toddler Maxine was told that her mother had died, she exclaimed, "I want to die too!"

Eugenia's husband, Uzell Ivy, age thirty-five, died that Saturday as well, passing at 3:10 AM in his father's home; Saturday was his father's 78th birthday. Eugenia and Uzell's son, Currie Ivy, age nine, showed no signs of illness Friday or Saturday morning. However, late Saturday afternoon, he fainted, dying one day later at 2:00 PM on Sunday.

Max Vunkannon, Myrtle's husband, age forty, passed away at 4:30 PM Saturday. Max's eighty-three-year-old father was traveling from Oregon by train to surprise his son for a visit at the time. He bought a newspaper at a stop in Mississippi and was shocked to read about his son's untimely death.

The last to succumb to the poison of botulinum toxin was Eugenia Ivy. Her death was slower than the rest. It's possible that she had a lower dose of the toxin. Eugenia felt ill Thursday evening after the meal and took chamomile tea and influenza medicine. Doctors thought that gave her a fighting chance to survive. The newspaper reported, "The same blindness which characterized the fatal illness of the other six victims attacked Mrs. Ivy also." She had paralysis of throat. The newspaper also reported that during Eugenia's last conscious moments she repeatedly moaned, "My husband is dead, and I have only my son to live for. If he dies, I want to die, too."

Unbeknownst to Eugenia, her nine-year-old son had already succumbed to botulism. Friends and physicians thought it was best to withhold the information of her son's death from her. When she inquired about him, she was told he was resting quietly. Eugenia Ivy, age thirty, died on Tuesday, February 10. Eugenia was buried next to her child, Currie Ivy, and her husband, Uzell Ivy, as well as Max Vunkannon, and his wife, Frances Myrtle Vunkannon. (Myrtle and Uzell were brother and sister).

In all, seven people died from the same olives that killed the victims of the Detroit outbreak and the Ohio outbreak. Mr. Alexander Stewart, the President of the Curtis Corporation, was "very indignant over the fact [that] the name of Curtis Corporation had been mentioned by the Memphis newspapers."

The clinical picture of botulism was becoming more detailed with each outbreak, but it was also becoming clearer to the medical profession that the variety of botulism symptoms was broader than commonly understood. The medical community began to realize, in retrospect, that many of the earlier food poisoning deaths attributed to ptomaine poisoning aligned with the symptoms of botulism.

In 1920, a medical journal article alerted physicians that in the previous six months there had been five botulism outbreaks from canned ripe olives tainted with botulinum toxin. Botulism outbreaks were frightening because they tended to bring swift deaths to family gatherings and could be caused by a variety of food sources. All commercially canned food became suspect, but consumers specifically avoided canned olives.

NEW REPORT IN OLIVE MYSTERY ALLEGES GERMAN CONSPIRACY TO POISON U. S. BOTTLED FOODS

"The aftermath of a gigantic German conspiracy to poison the bottled foods used in millions of American homes during the war, is the basis of a charge filed with the Department of Justice in Los Angeles today. This accusation has been filed as a result of a thorough investigation by packers into local methods of olive bottling following the recent deaths of botulinus poisoning reported in the east," reads an announcement received by The Telegram today.

"The fatalities in every instance were traced to olives bottled in glass. Olives packed in tin have constantly been immune from danger. The significant detail has just been discovered that all the poisonous glass jars, regardless of the firms bottling them, bore rubber ringed caps coming from a common source—a prominent eastern firm whose name is withheld from publication. Chemical analysis has divulged the fact that from these rubber caps, the necessary glycerin was deficient and therefore rendered the rubber caps leaky instead of airtight, with the consequent decomposition of the olives."

At a conference last week between ripe olive packers and health authorities of California, it was recommended that bottling of olives in glass jars hereafter be discontinued.

The Department of Justice is said to plan energetic steps to fathom the evil factors behind the alleged pernicious activity.

People were afraid to eat olives. Restaurants dropped olives from their menus. Housewives scratched olives off their shopping lists. In 1919, olive manufacturers enjoyed a $30,000,000 per year industry, only to see 95% of their market vanish due to the "great olive scare."

The rest of the canning industry watched as the momentum of public fear crippled the olive industry. Canners became worried that consumers might expand their suspicions and eventually reject all types of canned goods. The public was already suffering anxiety over food safety before the botulism outbreaks. In 1906, Upton Sinclair published *The Jungle*, a book written to expose the filth and lack of inspections in meat packing plants.

Olive canners were reluctant to take responsibility for their defective products. They generated theories that their products were poisoned by enemies of the state. When that theory failed to gain traction, they shifted the suspicion to the packers in the Midwest who bought their products in bulk at wholesale and repackaged them for consumer markets.

Finally, the industry tried to shift blame onto housewives by implying the safety of food was ultimately up to the housewife. She was expected to inspect every can of olives purchased and smell the contents for suspicious quality. While smelling canned food might have detected contents that were spoiled from decomposition, smelling would NOT be able to detect the presence of botulinum toxin, because it has no taste and no smell. Each attempt to shift blame was simply a corporate ploy to sidestep accountability.

Ultimately, it was the consumer reaction that held the canners responsible. Consumers quit believing the false advertisements in the newspapers assuring them that canned olives were safe to eat, and they simply stopped buying the product. Once consumers realized that botulinum toxin caused botulism, they wanted no part in it. The risk was simply too great. Eating olives was not a life-or-death necessity. This steep drop in market share drove the canners to eventually cooperate with the federal government and comply with safe canning practices as researched by Stanford University and Harvard University. Corporate malfeasance, then as it is now, was omnipresent in the marketplace.

TAKEAWAYS from
THE MEMPHIS, TENNESSEE OUTBREAK

Traditionally, corporations attempted to shift blame to consumers whenever their products caused harm or even wrongful deaths.

Unlike now, where food recalls happen quickly and even often voluntarily, corporations have historically tried to limit their liability by initially refusing to acknowledge even their potential liability.

In some cases, the victims with botulism knew they were going to die.

Botulism patients often underestimate their condition's severity; sudden decline and death can surprise both patient and physician.

Severity waxes and wanes. Victims have temporary improvements, then steep declines in status, resulting in fatal outcomes.

Complete respiratory collapse from botulism can happen with little to no warning, resulting in death within minutes.

CHAPTER 10

Pseudo Botulism Gaslighting
THE OAKLAND, CALIFORNIA
HOSPITAL OUTBREAK of 1920

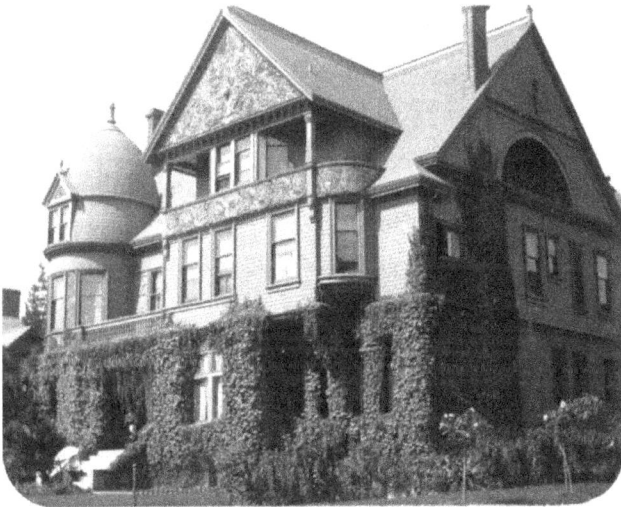

St. Anthony's Hospital, formerly the Edwin and Helen Goodall home built in 1880. Architect Walter Mathews.

Botulism outbreaks had become frightfully common by the 1920s even striking a hospital kitchen. On Thursday, October 14, 1920, St. Anthony's Hospital in Oakland, California served a noon meal to patients and staff that included canned spinach that unknowingly contained botulinum toxin.

Twelve people ate the spinach dish. Six people developed severe botulism, and three died. Additionally, who ate the spinach also showed acute symptoms of botulism, but they were diagnosed as having "pseudo botulism," implying that their illnesses were psychological. Granted, mild cases of botulism could be hard to diagnose, especially in isolation, but discounting the women's symptoms given the widespread nature of the botulism outbreak seems callous. Yet even in modern botulism outbreaks, undiagnosed botulism patients are misdiagnosed as hypochondriacs and suffering from a mental health condition.

The Chinese cook opened two cans of commercially packed spinach. He washed the spinach with cold tap water and placed it in a pan to bake in the oven for ten minutes. The odor from the cooking spinach permeated the kitchen, causing a nurse passing by to investigate. She traced the odor to the spinach; the cook acknowledged one of the cans was spoiled. At the nurse's suggestion, the cook removed the spoiled portion, opened a fresh can and added it into the pan, then continued to bake the dish. There were two issues with this food; it was of poor quality from decomposition and it contained botulinum toxin from improper canning procedures.

Two days after the spinach was consumed, the first symptoms appeared on Saturday, October 16. The original can and the contents were not available for inspection by the time the botulism outbreak was recognized. The *Oakland Tribune* captured how the botulism outbreak affected the people at the hospital:

> "Meanwhile grim terror stalks unhindered through the silent wards of the institution – fear is apparent on blanched faces of patients . . . as the knowledge that the attack of the pestilence is without warning. No one knows who the next victim will be."

On Tuesday evening, Dr. Geiger with the United States Public Health Department arrived on the scene. Dr. J.C. Geiger was a national authority on botulism and a member of the newly formed Botulism Commission. His comment to the press, while technically accurate, was not terribly assuring to the public: "The epidemic has been purely accidental and could not have been prevented by any member of the hospital staff. It might have happened in any hospital in the country."

Dr. Geiger was critical of the hospital staff for missing what he felt was an obvious diagnosis. He said, "The symptoms were typical from the onset, and diagnosis should have been comparatively easy." Even a botulism outbreak in a hospital setting evaded an accurate and timely diagnosis. Recognizing botulism was easy for someone versed in the symptomatology of botulism, but seemingly impossible for a medical staff unfamiliar with the disease.

Once Dr. Geiger informed the hospital of botulism, staff tracked discharged patients and monitored for the next victim of a poison that could progress rapidly or insidiously slowly.

The newspaper explained, "Adding to the horror of the intangible enemy, came the word from medical experts that it often took from twenty-four to forty-eight hours for the poison, should it prove to be botulism, to take effect."

The Fatal Cases

Dr. Edith Strong had been employed by the St. Anthony's Hospital for almost one year. Previously, she was a practicing MD in St. Louis, Missouri. She earned her medical degree in St. Louis in 1907. (Ironically, two days before her death, she had made out a legal will that specified her automobile proceeds, life insurance proceeds, and $700 of assets should go to Miss Jenny Mahoney for the maintenance of her two cats.) Dr. Strong complained of feeling ill on Tuesday. She was placed under medical attention and lost consciousness. Respiration was poor. She died within two hours while still unconscious. Edith Josephine Strong, age forty-nine, died on Tuesday, October 19, five days after ingesting botulinum toxin.

Anna Renas worked as a nurse for ten years at St. Anthony's Hospital. She lived in Oakley, California but was a native of Antioch. During her botulism illness, she lapsed into "long intervals of unconsciousness." Later the doctors thought the course of her illness had changed for the better and believed she had a chance at recovery.

Anna Kennedy Renas, age thirty-four, died on Sunday, October 17, three days after ingesting botulinum toxin.

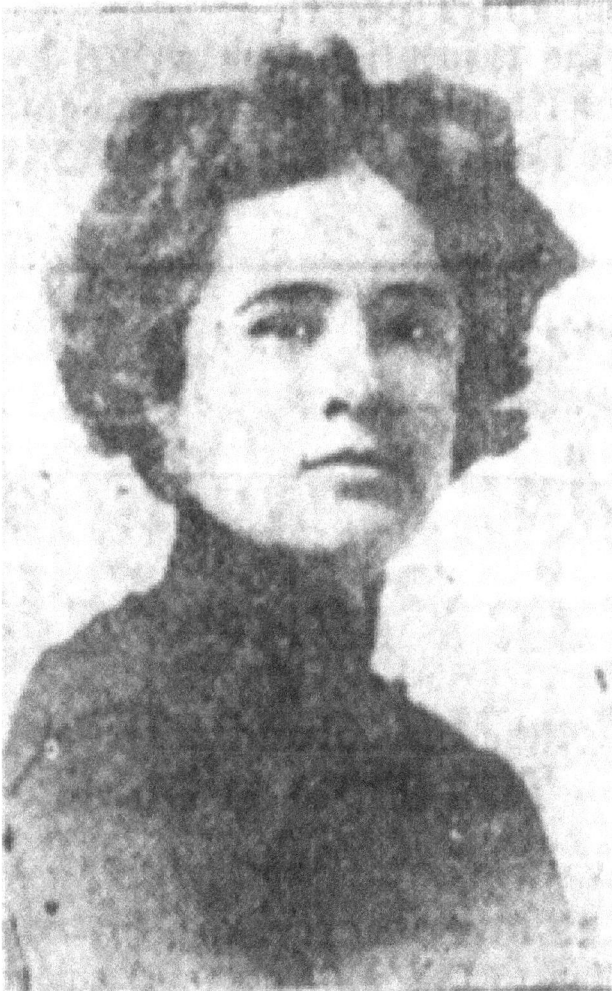

Anna Kennedy Renas

The final fatality was Joseph Freitas, who was a patient at St. Anthony's Hospital. He had been treated for a broken arm and released, but returned later complaining of illness. He died shortly after he was readmitted to the hospital. The botulism antitoxin had not arrived in time to administer to him. Joseph Freitas, age thirty-seven, died Wednesday, October 20, six days after ingesting botulinum toxin.

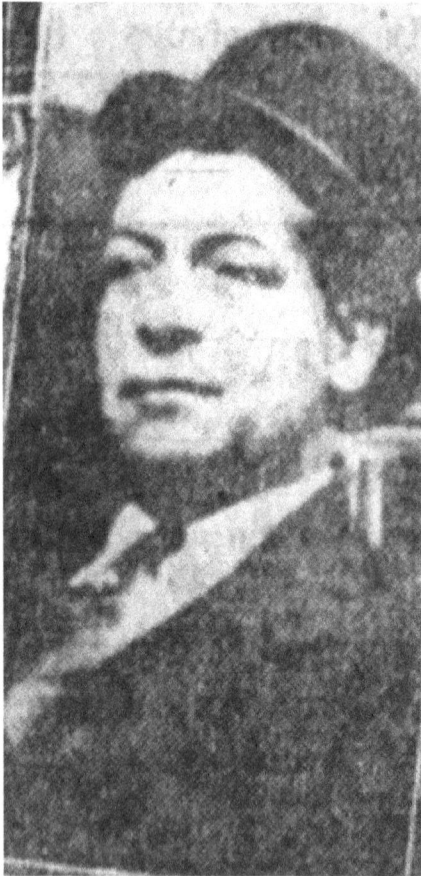

Joseph Freitas

The Surviving Cases

A victim with a mild case of botulism, identified only as "J.M." in the medical reports, was not discovered until October 23, a full nine days after ingestion of the toxin occurred. J.M. was hospitalized in San Francisco, but not given the antitoxin. He recovered. Two additional poisoning victims were fortunate enough to be given the antitoxin: Nellie F. Russell, a private nurse, and Steven Wendt, a patient also treated for a broken arm. Both survived. This was the first use of the experimental antitoxin developed by The Botulism Commission. Seven-hundred and fifty guinea pigs were used in the development of the antitoxins for botulinum toxin type A and type B.

Because Nellie Russell's case was so severe and she was not predicted to live, Dr. Geiger wrote a detailed case report on the progress of her illness and response to the botulism antitoxin. On Tuesday, October 19, Nellie had extreme difficulty in breathing, swallowing, and speech. She had a distressing cough and was not able to remove the mucus stuck in her throat. She had ptosis in the left eyelid. She also had double vision. Nellie experienced extreme weakness, particularly when trying to lift or hold up her head. Her pulse was rapid and body temperature was subnormal. She was apprehensive, but had no pain and no worry. When Dr. Geiger examined Nellie, he reported she "had every clinical sign predicting a fatal termination."

The botulism antitoxin was administered to Nellie on three consecutive days. She showed massive improvement four hours after the second dose. Most of the symptoms improved except her vision, which remained impaired. Dr. Geiger noted that throughout the recovery a "rather violent erythema still persisted." Erythema is an abnormal redness of the skin and considered an atypical symptom of botulism.

TAKEAWAYS from
THE OAKLAND, CALIFORNIA, OUTBREAK

Individual cases of botulism are routinely misdiagnosed.

Within a single botulism outbreak, patients can share some symptoms in common, but can also present with a different combination of symptoms from one another.

The concerns of female patients who reported symptoms of botulism were ridiculed.

Medical professionals missed obvious neurological symptoms in their patients and in themselves that were indicative of botulism.

Botulism patients often underestimate their condition's severity; sudden decline and death can surprise both patient and physician.

Complete respiratory collapse from botulism can happen with little to no warning, resulting in death within minutes.

CHAPTER 11

Dead Wrong: Friends Assume Safety
THE GREENSBURG, PENNSYLVANIA,
OUTBREAK of 1921

The Wentling family tradition was to celebrate birthdays with a dinner for family and friends. For Joseph Wentling's forty-fifth birthday, his wife, Mary, arranged a lovely picnic at a popular amusement park, Oakford Park in nearby Jeannette, Pennsylvania. This trolley park hosted as many as 20,000 visitors per day. The trolley shuttled patrons from Greensburg straight to Oakford Park in Jeannette, five miles away. Oakford Park featured a miniature railway ride, a rollercoaster, a penny arcade, a merry-go-round, a picnic shed, a cottage for ladies, a dance hall, a laughing gallery, a 5¢ movie theater, a skating rink, and a bandstand for live entertainment. Oakford Park was a source of never-ending fun for the community. Joseph, Mary, and their nursemaid provided the five Wentling children with one last day of family memories.

June 21, 1921 resulted in unthinkable tragedy for the Wentling party. Of the eight guests, three would die of botulism. One of the fatal cases was Mary Wentling, age thirty-nine, who was five months pregnant at the time of death. Another fatal case was the nursemaid who cared for the five young Wentling children. Within two days, the Wentling children lost the two most important women in their lives: their mother and their nursemaid. Plus, Joseph Wentling lost his sister.

When Mary Lynch was twenty-five, she began her life with attorney Joseph D. Wentling, age thirty-one, on May 15, 1907. Mary was the daughter of Thomas Lynch, the president of H.C. Frick Coke company. The bride's family hosted a wedding at the Lynch estate in Greensburg, Pennsylvania. The reception that followed included four hundred guests.

After a month-long honeymoon, Mary and Joseph settled down in a stately two-story brick home on Seminary Avenue near the Lynch estate. Together, Mary and Joseph brought five children into the world: Nancy in 1908, Sally in 1912, Joseph Jr. in 1914, Thomas in 1916, and Mary in 1917. Their sixth child was due in the fall of 1921.

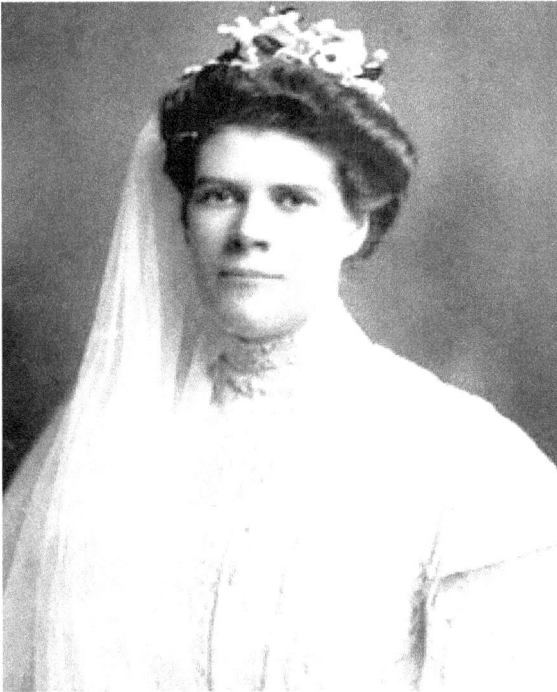

Mary Lynch Wentling

The Wentlings were well known in the Greensburg community of fifteen-thousand residents. The newspapers described Joseph and Mary Wentling as being "prominently identified with civic and charitable undertakings" and playing significant parts in the war drives.

The Wentling birthday party was held on Tuesday, June 21, 1921, and included Joseph's sisters: Mercedes "Goldie" Wentling and Harriet "Hydie" Wentling Reed along with her husband, John Covode Reed. Other attendees included Harry and Mary Bovard. The Wentling children invited three of their playmates from the Jamison family to the park: Priscilla, age twelve; Elizabeth, age eleven, and Thomas, age nine. Ironically, Jamison children had lost their mother to cancer in 1916 so Mary included the children in the Wentling family events.

Toward the end of the outing, the children were allowed to remain in the park to eat their supper there with the nursemaid, as they did not mind the heat so much. The adult guests returned to the Wentling home, bringing with them some of the picnic lunch, including the olives. At 7:00 PM, the meal at the Wentling home included cantaloupe, boiled spring chicken, potatoes with butter sauce, new peas from the Wentling garden, stuffed fresh tomatoes with rice, lettuce salad, ice cream, coffee, cake–and ripe olives.

It was the ripe olives that gave pause to one of the guests. Hydie Reed remarked that the olives served were the first she had considered eating since the tragedy that befell her friends in Detroit, Michigan, two years prior. Hydie knew the Sales family from Grosse Pointe, Michigan, and recalled the fatal outcomes of that botulism outbreak in 1919. (The Sales served olives at a dinner party that resulted in the death of two of their children, two maids, and a dear friend.) Mary Wentling assured Hydie that there was no reason to be alarmed and stated, "We have had this brand before." Mary and Hydie decided to serve the olives at the party.

Joseph and Mary Wentling had purchased the olives in January 1921 and saved them for six months for use in a special occasion. The canning industry had also issued press releases that improvements had been made in canning procedures and reassured the public that olives were, once again, safe to eat. Unbeknownst to the Wentlings, the olives they purchased had been packed in April 1920 at a time when the fruit packers were still adapting to the new food safety science canning recommendation and attempting to comply with new inspections by government agencies. Compliance proved difficult as many instances of fraudulent records were discovered by the inspectors.

The Wentlings employed a nursemaid, Ethel Woodward, who had been with the family for fifteen years. She cared for the children, ages three, five, seven, nine, and thirteen

When Ethel returned home from the park with the children, she also ate three olives Tuesday evening and three more Wednesday morning. She vomited on Thursday and was reported as "seriously ill and her condition became critical almost at once." Ethel was having trouble breathing to the point of turning "blue, threshing about on the bed and grabbing at her neck." She experienced convulsions shortly before her death at noon on Thursday, June 23, 1921. Her pulse continued for two minutes after respiration failed. Ethel Woodward, age thirty-two, was a hearty woman weighing 240 pounds at the time of her death. Though the doctors noted Ethel's weight, botulinum toxin is equally lethal to a small child or a large adult because it acts on the neuromuscular junctions to cause flaccid paralysis resulting in fatal respiratory failure or cardiac deaths.

Mary Wentling's first symptom of illness appeared on Wednesday just one day after the birthday party. She became nauseated after eating a tomato sandwich at the country club and immediately returned home. She vomited at 1:30 AM and was treated for gastrointestinal distress by her physician. She felt better until noon Thursday when she developed a slight difficulty in articulation and then vomited again. By 3:00 PM, Mary's articulation progressively worsened and her respiration became difficult. Her condition grew more and more critical with each passing moment. Her heart rate was 156 beats per minute. At no time did she have any facial paralysis. Mary Lynch Wentling, age thirty-nine, suddenly died of respiratory paralysis at 10:00 PM on Thursday, June 23. She left behind her husband and five children; her fetus perished as well.

Joseph Wentling was stunned by the unfolding tragedy that resulted in two deaths in the household on Thursday. When investigated, he could not recall what food items were consumed at his birthday celebration. The two Slavish maids in the kitchen became very frightened over witnessing the illnesses and deaths. One maid had tasted an olive and not liking the taste, spat it out. Another maid was described as "temporarily insane" from the ordeal.

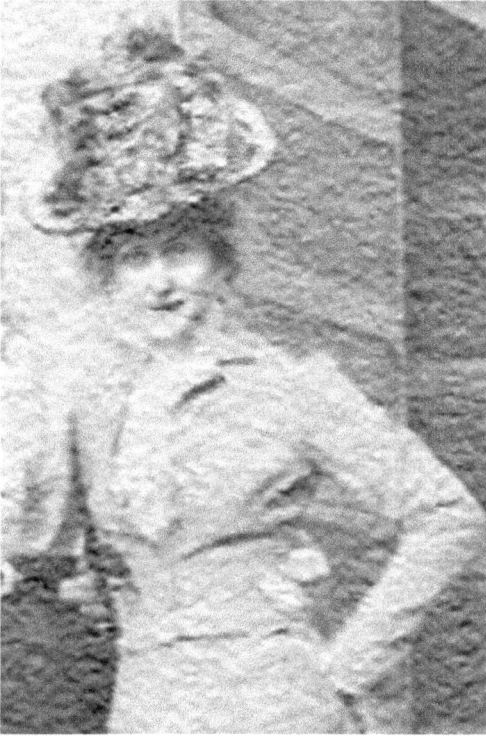

Hydie (Wentling) Reed

Hydie Reed, Joseph's older sister, had eaten only one or two olives. She showed no signs of poisoning until Thursday morning. She complained of a dry throat and had difficulty articulating her words. She did not have the typical symptom of vomiting, nor did she have a headache. Thirty-six hours after she ate the two olives, she had double vision and blurry vision. After sixty hours, her body was turning blue from lack of oxygen. After sixty-four hours, she could not swallow her own saliva. She also had ptosis of both eyelids. However, she presented an atypical symptom of botulism–anuria, a failure of the kidneys to produce urine.

Her physicians recalled reading an article just a few days earlier about the use of anesthesia in evaluating the toxicity of botulinum toxin in animal experiments. The June 18th article in the Journal of the American Medical Association postulated that by anesthetizing the patient, the nerves might heal and allow for normal breathing to resume. This experimental treatment was initiated on Hydie on Friday, June 24, 1921.

The antitoxin also arrived on Friday and was administered to Hydie Reed in two doses. Though still critical, Hydie had a slight change in her condition, and the newspapers reported "hope was given that she had passed the crisis." As a desperate medical intervention, Hydie was placed under anesthetic for the last three days of her life, an action that we now know likely prevented any chance of her survival. Harriet "Hydie" (Wentling) Reed, age forty-six, did not survive her encounter with botulinum toxin and died on Monday, June 27.

Survivors of Botulism

Goldie Wentling, Joseph's younger sister, had eaten quite heartily of the olives. Before going home, she drank one beer at the invitation of her brother. Once at home, Goldie became nauseated and vomited. The newspapers speculated that because her stomach contents were purged, she might have escaped a fatal outcome from the poisoning. Though Prohibition of alcohol was still in effect, not much attention was focused Goldie's one beer after the celebration.

Goldie collapsed on Sunday after being in constant attendance at the bedside of Hydie, her dying sister. At no time was Goldie's condition considered nearly as serious as the others. One doctor thought Goldie's troubles were from exhaustion and nervousness while the other doctor believed Goldie had mild symptoms of botulism.

Mary Bovard said she ate only one olive, which she described as large and delicious. Mary said she would have eaten more, but the dish of olives was at the other end of the table, and she did not ask for it to be passed. That decision spared her life. She may have been saving the delicacy for the immediate family to enjoy. After all, this was a family celebration and she was a guest.

Later during the investigation, the olives in question from the Wentling dinner were determined to contain botulinum toxin. Testing the poison on chickens was a simple and accessible test. The olives were fed to two chickens. The first chicken developed a condition called *limberneck* and died within thirty-six hours, and the second chicken became groggy. Both chickens presented with telltale signs of botulism.

The irony of this botulism outbreak is how preventable it was. Olive recalls had been in the newspapers for two years. There were multiple deaths from olives tainted with botulinum toxin reported from coast to coast. The women hosting the party personally knew about the lethality of botulinum toxin, but they assumed the product in their hands was safe. Somehow death was something that happened to other people but not them? The women knew that the prudent course of action would be to forego the olives and yet the hostess assumed there were no risks. They were dead wrong.

By 1921, the olive packers had become creative about their enticements to regain their lost markets. They hid a $20 gold piece in a can of olives, worth about $350 in 2025 dollars.

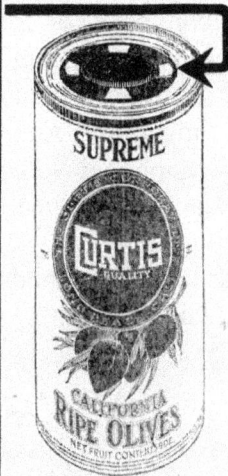

Eventually, the Wentling children had a happy ending to this tragic experience. Their father, Joseph, telephoned his parents for recommendations on hired help. They offered their trusted household helper, Anna O'Hara, who had served as a Red Cross nurse in the Great War.

However, an unmarried woman living in a home with a widowed man and his children appeared socially inappropriate for a family of the Wentling's stature. The solution was simple. In 1923, Joseph Wentling and Anna

O'Hara were married, and together they raised the five children in the home at 135 Seminary Avenue in Greensburg. What was initially a marriage of convenience for appearance's sake became a genuine marriage based on love. Family folklore reveals that the children thought of Anna O'Hara like a mother and remained devoted to her until her untimely death from a heart attack in 1945.

The Wentling red-brick home still stands today in historic downtown Greensburg.

TAKEAWAYS from
THE GREENSBURG OUTBREAK

Medical professionals discounted the female patients when they reported concerns or mild symptoms.

The chickens that were fed the food tainted with botulinum toxin died of botulism.

Atypical symptoms routinely occur in botulism cases where details are captured. In this case, the ability to urinate was affected.

There is variability in the symptoms even within the same botulism outbreak.
\
Severity waxes and wanes. Victims have temporary improvements, then steep declines in status, resulting in fatal outcomes.

Convulsions prior to death from botulinum toxin entering the brain are commonly reported, but not widely known.

Consumers believed assurances from corporations that their products were safe when, in fact, the corporations blatantly ignored scientific evidence and prioritized profits above the consumers' safety.

CHAPTER 12

A Reunion with Death
THE ALBANY, OREGON
OUTBREAK of 1924

One of the largest botulism outbreaks in U.S. history occurred in Albany, Oregon, and had a 100% fatality rate that claimed the lives of twelve people. On February 2, 1924, four German families came together in celebration for a family reunion. The Gerbers and Gerbigs hosted a welcome dinner for Paul Gerbig, Sr.'s daughter Paula Ruehling and her husband, Curt, and their baby, Horst. The Ruehlings had recently arrived in the United States from Germany. Curt had been a soldier in the German army in the Great War.

Emilie Gerber, or Grandmother Gerber, as the family called her, had grown a garden and canned food for thirty years. Her home was stockpiled full of her home-canned produce. She was an "experienced packer" who had sold her home-canned goods to neighbors for years. *The Albany Daily Democrat* reported:

"Her food products had such a good reputation in the neighborhood that the friends used to beg her for a few jars of some favorite fruit or vegetable. The string beans were so much admired that on the occasion of this family reunion one of the mothers fed a nursing baby with a teaspoon of the juice and another started off her nursing with a string bean on which to chew as a pacifier."

The green beans in question served at the reunion were used in a cold wax bean salad. They had been canned two years prior to the meal. After the tragedy, the family recalled an episode of limberneck chickens that died from contaminated food stock around the same time as this batch of green beans was home-canned by Grandmother Gerber.

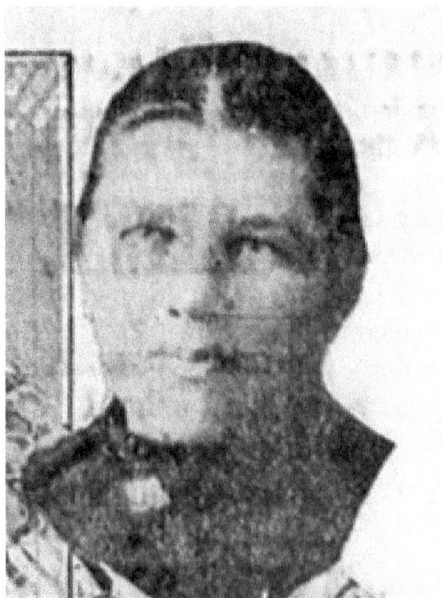

Emilie (Yunker) Gerber

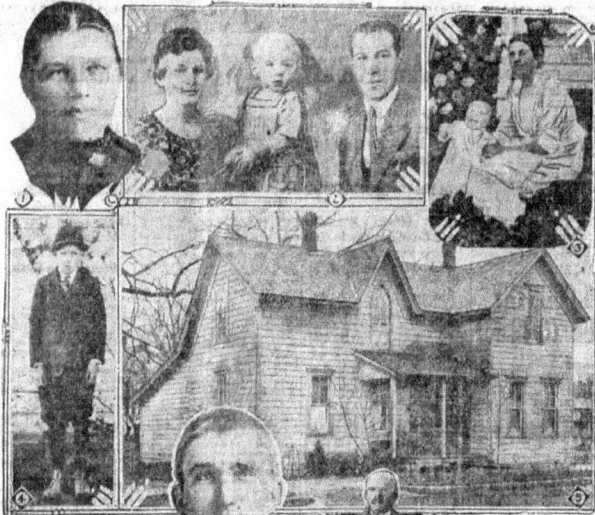

FOUR FAMILIES HIT BY POISONING TRAGEDY

—Courtesy of Portland Telegram

No. 1—Mrs. Reinhold Gerber, hostess at the fatal family reunion dinner which resulted in 11 deaths and one fatal illness. No. 2—Mr. and Mrs. Kurt Ruehling, dead, and two-year-old son Horst, dying. No. 3—Mrs. Paul Gerbig and 10 months-old daughter, father, who lies beside her mother in the same casket. No. 4—Hans Yunker, nephew of Mrs. Gerber, whose mother and brother by a stroke of fortune were not at the dinner. No. 5 —Gerber home at 814 Baker street, where the feast of death was served. No. 6—Paul Gerbig, whose family has been obliterated. No. 7—Reinhold Gerber, father of Mrs. Paul Gerbig.

BOTULINE STOR
TOLD BY STA
HEALTH OFFIC

By Dr. Frederick D. Stricke
Botulism is a deadly food p
The name botulism has lost its
al significance which was sa
poisoning. It was thought the
germ that produces the poison
ing botulism would grow only in

Gerber home at 814 Baker Street, Albany, Oregon, is
still standing today as a historic property.

The Fatal Cases

1. Emilie (Yunker) Gerber, age 70
   (Reinhold's wife)
2. Reinhold Gerber, age 73
   (Emilie's husband)
3. Margaret Gerbig, age 34
   (daughter of Emilie and Reinhold)
4. Paul Otto Gerbig, age 35
   (Margaret's husband)
5. Hilda Gerbig, age 10
   (child of Margaret and Paul)
6. Marie Gerbig, age 7
   (child of Margaret and Paul)
7. Margareth Gerbig, age 5
   (child of Margaret and Paul)
8. Esther Gerbig, age 13 months
   (child of Margaret and Paul)
9. Hans Yunker, 12
   (Emilie and Reinhold's nephew)
10. Paula Ruehling, age 23
    (Paul Gerbig's sister)
11. Gottfried (aka Curt) Ruehling, age 25
    (Paula's husband)
12. Horst Ruehling, 18 months
    (Paula and Curt's child)

The case report detailed the maladies of the botulism patients, which, at times, did not appear serious or potentially fatal. Some of the sick victims exhibited a stamina uncharacteristic of patients weakened from botulism. The victims did not suspect their deaths were imminent. This surge of energy mystified physicians and led all involved to underestimate the seriousness of the situation.

"Five of the cases [out of 12] could be considered ambulatory, as they remained up and moving about almost until the time of death. In fact, one case took excellent care of several others, notwithstanding the fact that the symptoms of difficulty in vision, respiration, and swallowing, and in the presence of a large amount of mucus in the throat, were constantly present. Another case drove an automobile several times on the trip from Albany to the country ranch and return."

Eleven of the victims died quickly, within one to four days of ingesting the botulinum toxin-laden beans. One lingered for a week. As a lot, they were "restless and apprehensive." The neurological symptoms varied, but most had double vision and muscle weakness all over. Nausea was common. Ten of the twelve vomited. Four of the twelve experienced ptosis, the swollen eyelids. Three of the twelve displayed tremors. Two of the twelve had limbs that were completely paralyzed. One had diarrhea, but then became constipated. The nerves in the bowel become damaged and are no longer able to hold the feces. Shortly thereafter, the digestive track becomes paralyzed and unable to move the bowels. Three of the twelve were unconscious before death, and one of those cases was marked by "agonizing pain." Two cases were progressing favorably, then rapidly became worse after they were fed a hearty meal.

The newspaper reported though not the first to die, the first to fall ill was the Gerbig's son-in-law, Paul. The story described the unique features of his demise:

"Paul Gerbig, whose marvelous constitution had enabled him to withstand the ravages of the poison longer than all the rest, finally yielded his life at 9:30 o'clock. But Paul Gerbig paid for his four-day battle with death. The end came amid agonizing convulsions and pain such as few of those who had preceded him had suffered."

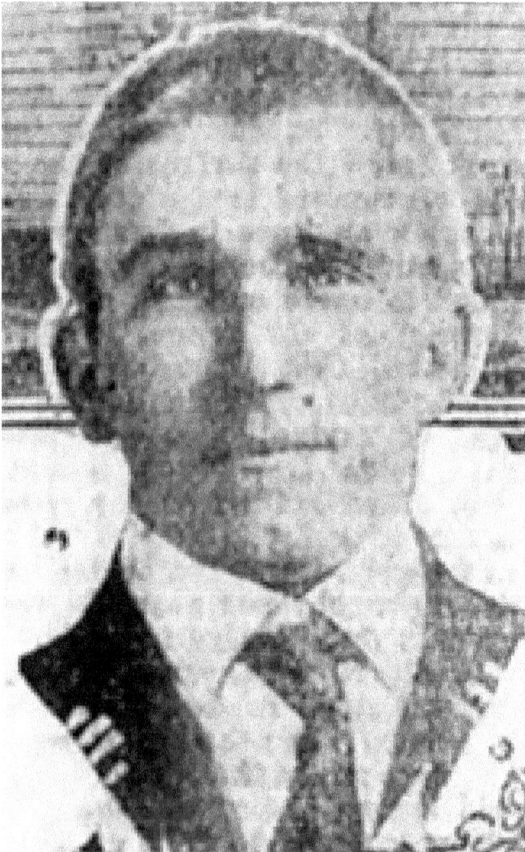

Paul Gerbig

The last to die was the baby, Horst Ruehling. Prior to his death, the newspapers referred to the orphaned German infant as "the homeless baby." The newspaper stated:

> "Assurance was given today the Lutheran church congregation will see to it that he shall never want for parents. A thousand homes in Linn County are ready to receive him."

On the fourth day after the meal, Horst was described as "blithesome and gay, seemingly untouched by the deadly venom." He was expected to survive, but on the fifth day, the newspaper reported his condition deteriorated quickly:

> "He was intermittently in a stupor. Sometimes he would cry. Sometimes he would feel better. Then would come semi consciousness, again. But still he lives. Until late last night, it was believed certain that the little boy had escaped poisoning, despite the fact that he had partaken of the venomous beans at the Gerber family reunion Saturday noon.
>
> He had been slightly ill, it is true, but had shown no symptoms such as had rendered him an orphan and without relatives in America. At 8 o'clock he began acting as had the rest. He evinced a tendency to choke when given water to drink. These symptoms continued more marked today. Although he was still able to be around, and to play a little. This afternoon his steps were lagging and it was deemed only a matter of a

few hours or a few days until he will follow the rest."

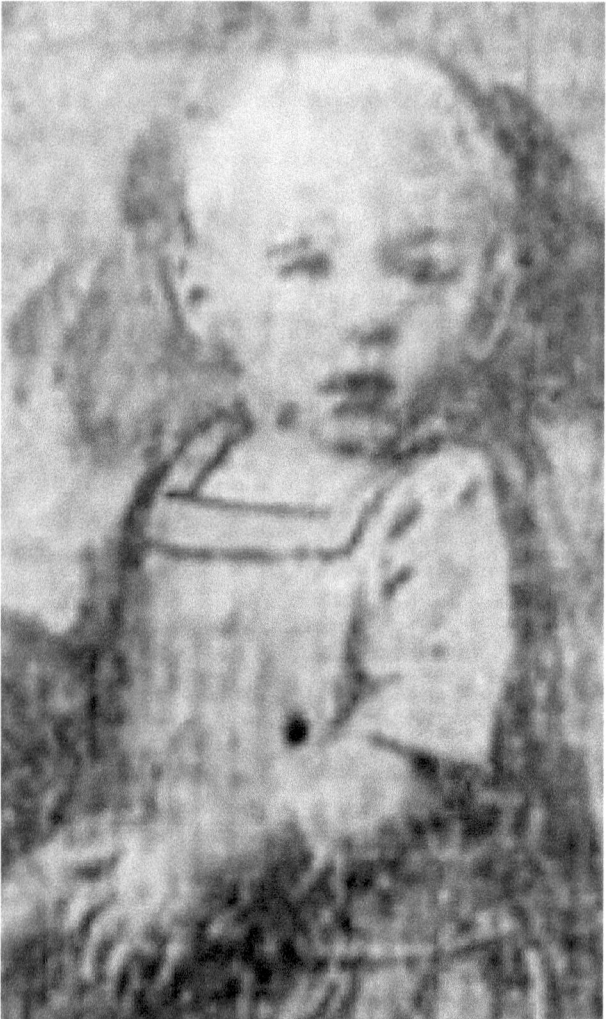

Horst Ruehling

An experimental botulism antitoxin serum had arrived in Albany five days after Horst Ruehling ingested the poison, but it was determined that the poison had "already made too much progress to permit such treatment and an injection under the circumstances might only bring instant death."

The physicians wrongly assumed the antitoxin serum had only been used experimentally on animals up to this point, and administration to the young boy would have been "merely experimental" and "without the smallest hope for success."

Even a delayed administration of the botulism antitoxin likely would have saved the life of the child. In this case, the botulism antitoxin was withheld from the child on the fifth day after ingesting botulinum toxin. Even in the 1920s, research proved the toxin was still circulating in the bloodstream after fourteen days; however, such research might have been difficult to locate in the midst of a chaotic outbreak.

A mass funeral for the eleven dead was held at the First Presbyterian Church attended by fifteen hundred people from the community while hundreds more stood outside in mourning on a cold February day. A twelfth coffin, child-sized, was prepared at the Fisher-Braden funeral parlor in anticipation of the Ruehling toddler who was teetering between life and death at the time of the funerals. Horst Ruehling died on the eighth day after the poisoning and was buried next to his parents after a private graveside ceremony.

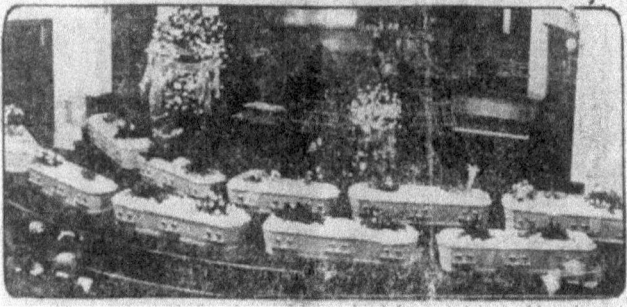

BURIAL OF ELEVEN POISON VICTIMS

In the funeral congregation were Mr. and Mrs. Yunker and their five children: Werner, Carl, Gertrude, Otto Jr., and Alfred. Grandmother Gerber's maiden name was Yunker. Mr. Yunker had dropped off Hans Yunker at the Gerber reunion dinner and gone back to the Yunker home to pick up more family to attend. Car trouble kept them from returning to the reunion that day. Meanwhile, young Hans Yunker ate the toxic green beans and later died from botulism along with the rest of his aunt's family. Local photographer Clarence Clifford memorialized the funeral scene in still images. The Oregon Journal's reporter F.C. Heath captured film footage of the event and made a newsreel to show in the motion picture theaters.

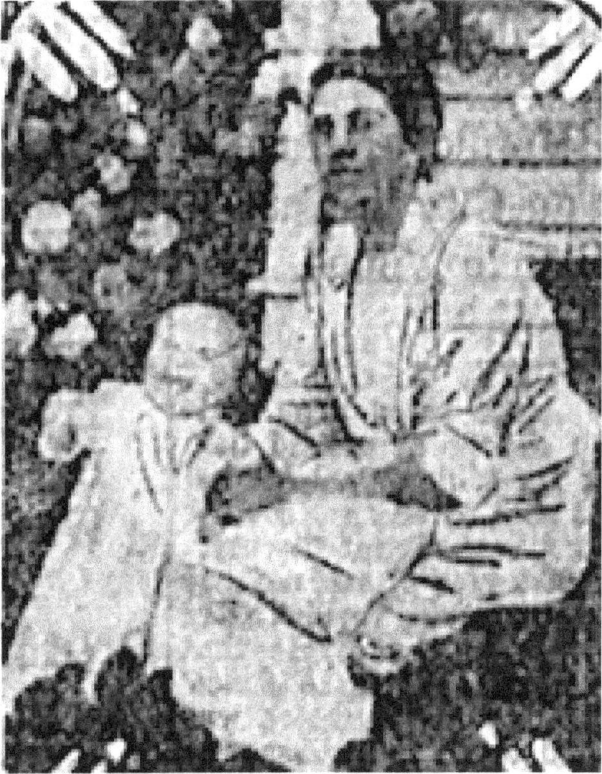

13-month-old Esther was placed next to her
mother in the mother's casket

Thirteen days after the fateful reunion dinner,
investigators were surprised to find the green beans
served at the family reunion dinner scattered about
on the ground outside the Gerber home. It was
common practice to feed table scraps to the animals
outside. These beans suspected as the source of
poison were tested and found to still have high
levels of botulinum toxin in them, even thirteen
days after the dinner. Also, investigators discovered
that the soil in the vegetable garden was saturated
with the *Clostridium botulinum* spores, the spores

being the original source of the toxin. An additional five jars of unopened canned green beans from the same pack were found in the Gerber's pantry. Visually, the green beans were "normal in appearance and odor" yet tested positive for botulinum toxin, enough, in fact, to "do away with the entire community" warned the newspapers. What may have sounded like a wild exaggeration by the public health scientists, likely wasn't. By 1922, the professors at Harvard University had determined that ONE drop of botulinum toxin would kill every human being on Earth, or two billion people.

Two autopsies were performed and a treatment of botulism antitoxin was provided to the doctors to use in case they developed symptoms of botulism from attending the dying and dead. It was unclear at the time if botulinum toxin could be transmitted through an open skin abrasion that came in contact with bodily fluids from a botulism patient. This was a wise precautionary decision.

TAKEAWAYS from
THE ALBANY, OREGON, OUTBREAK

Botulism patients often underestimate their condition's severity; sudden decline and death can surprise both patient and physician.

There is variability in the symptoms even within the same botulism outbreak.

Complete respiratory collapse from botulism can happen with little to no warning, resulting in death within minutes.

Convulsions prior to death from botulinum toxin entering the brain are commonly reported, but not widely known.

Botulism symptoms wax and wane, giving hope for recovery, only to suddenly result in a fatal outcome.

Delayed administration of the antitoxin contributed to a fatal outcome.

CHAPTER 13

Mild Botulism Can Also be Fatal
THE GRAFTON, NORTH DAKOTA
OUTBREAK of 1931

On January 29, 1931, seventeen partygoers gathered at the Hein farm, located two miles northeast of Grafton, North Dakota, to celebrate a "midnight lunch" and break the monotony of a harsh winter night. The festivities–complete with food, drinks, dancing, and games–offered a respite from the isolation of North Dakota winters. However, the evening took a tragic turn when botulinum toxin, unknowingly present in a jar of home-canned peas, led to the deaths of thirteen attendees. The devastating outbreak of botulism shocked the small rural community and sent ripples of horror throughout the state, marking one of the most tragic incidents in North Dakota's history.

In 1931, Grafton, North Dakota, was a quiet town of about three thousand residents, nestled less than fifty miles south of the Canadian border. That winter, Edward and Delphine Hein invited friends and neighbors to their home for their annual "midnight lunch" party, a cherished tradition in the rural community. The event was meant to be a celebration of warmth and camaraderie—an antidote to the cold and harsh North Dakota winter. However, what began as a joyful gathering turned into a tragedy of unfathomable scale. The deaths of thirteen partygoers sent an overwhelming grief through the tight-knit farming community, leaving an indelible mark on the region that would resonate for generations.

The Heins had invited over fifty people to their annual gathering, a tradition that typically drew many from the rural community. However, on this particular evening, poor weather, snow drifts, and a competing event in Grafton had limited the attendance and only about twenty people showed up to the party. One couple was delayed by a snowdrift and ultimately had to turn back, while others were similarly deterred by the weather.

The Heins' three youngest children Richard, age fourteen, Wilfred, age twelve, and Marvin (Buddy), age four, were too young to join the late-night festivities, so they remained safely asleep in their beds. Meanwhile, their three older siblings attended the party, unaware that it would be their last. The tragedy that followed would forever alter the course of the Hein family and their community.

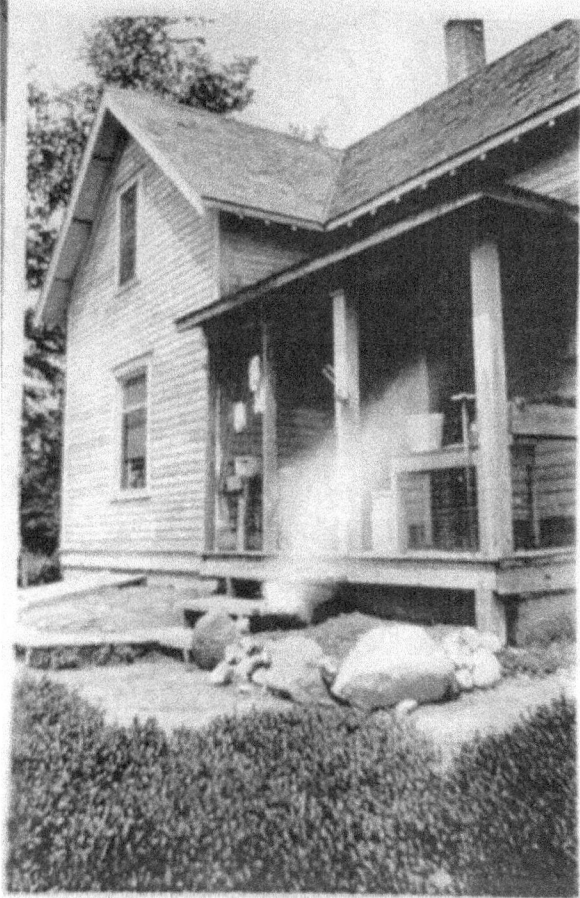

The Heins' yellow farmhouse northeast of
Grafton, North Dakota

Delphine Hein served coffee, buns, hot boiled
wieners, light spice cake, and a vegetable salad
made with home-canned vegetables (carrots, peas,
and cut string beans) with a whipped cream
dressing and served on lettuce. Home-canned peas
were the suspected source of botulinum toxin. The
medical report stated:

"Sixteen of the seventeen present partook of the entire lunch, one guest declining to eat the salad because he never ate vegetables in any form, subsequently he did not become ill. Thirteen of the sixteen who ate the salad afterwards became ill and died. The remaining three who ate the salad and did not subsequently become ill therefrom were intoxicated at the time of eating, had been nauseated and vomited before lunch was served and vomited again during or just after lunch. "Moon" or "hootch," homemade beer, and wine for the liquors were consumed by several who attended the party."

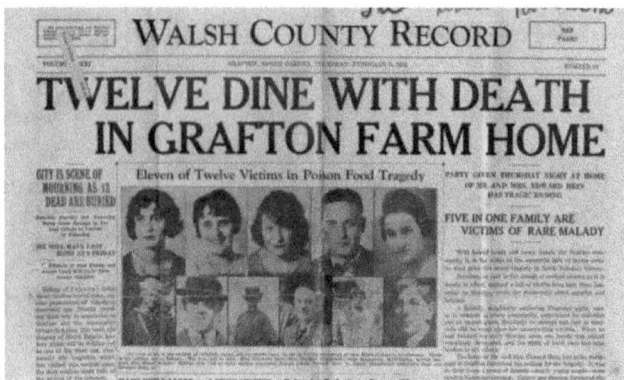

WALSH COUNTY RECORD

TWELVE DINE WITH DEATH IN GRAFTON FARM HOME

Eleven of Twelve Victims in Poison Food Tragedy

The botulism outbreak in Grafton sent shockwaves across the country, already reeling from the hardships of the Great Depression. Home-canned goods had become a reliable staple in hard economic times. The victims of this devastating tragedy included members of several families and friends: the Hein family, which lost a mother, father, three children, and a cousin; the Chapiewski family, which lost a mother and her son; the

Lessard family, which mourned the loss of two relatives; and three other unrelated local friends. The scale of the tragedy, coupled with the overwhelming grief of a community already struggling, made the outbreak all the more harrowing.

Arthur Jorandby was recorded as the first death, though technically others died earlier. A native of Grafton, Arthur graduated from Grafton High School in 1918 and, soon after, enlisted in the U.S. Navy. He served aboard the U.S.S. Rijndam in France during the Great War, achieving the rank of seaman second class. After the war, Arthur returned to Grafton to help his father manage the family's extensive farming operations. Arthur became a well-known and respected member of the community. His untimely death would mark the beginning of a devastating outbreak that would touch countless lives.

After the Thursday night party at the Hein farm, Arthur worked with his father on the farm all day Friday. That evening by 9:30 PM Arthur told his brother George that he felt dizzy, but he did not consider his ailment serious and retired to bed. He woke up at 11:30 PM and told his brother that he was feeling worse and had "awful pains" in his stomach. A doctor was summoned to the house immediately. Arthur fell into a coma for 15 hours. Just before his death he complained of gripping pains in his stomach, chest, and lungs. Arthur Elliot Jorandby, age thirty-two, died at 3:30 PM on Saturday, January 31. The treating physician immediately and accurately diagnosed the death as a case of botulism based on several medical publications on botulism outbreaks that he had read.

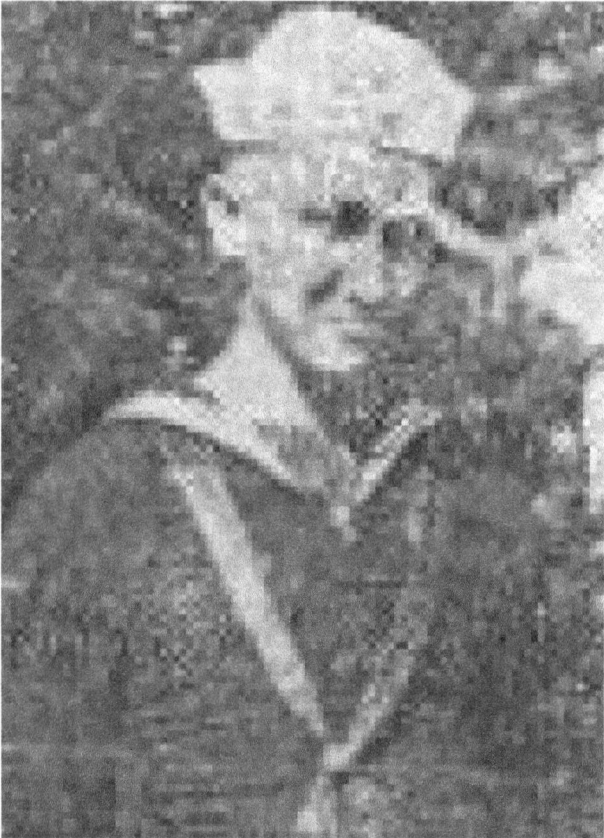

Arthur Elliot Jorandby

The wave of death continued to sweep through the community and affected the households of the Heins and Chapiewskis next. They were unaware of the tragedy that had already claimed Arthur Jorandby's life. Harry Chapiewski, the youngest victim, was an up-and-coming star on his high school basketball team. On the afternoon of Friday,

January 30, he attended classes, and later that evening, he played in a practice game. Afterward, he returned home to find his parents, Bebe Anna and Edward Chapiewski, hosting Angeline and Elmer Stokke for dinner, a frequent gathering in the Chapiewski home.

That evening, Angeline Stokke mentioned having a headache, though she thought little of it since she often suffered from them. Hours later, Harry's mother, Bebe Anna, began to complain of a similar headache. By the next day, Harry suddenly had fallen ill, and his condition quickly worsened. The rapid onset of symptoms in the Chapiewski household foreshadowed the tragic toll the outbreak would take. Harold J. Chapiewski, age sixteen, died at 6:10 PM on Saturday, January 31.

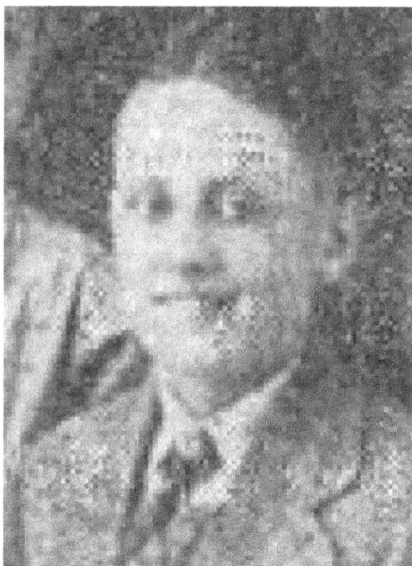

Harry Chapiewski

Bebe Anna married Thomas Chapiewski in 1912, and the couple moved to Grafton when Thomas took a job at the Berg & Flekke Store. In 1927, Thomas purchased the Grafton Café, and the family settled into a new phase of life. Thomas did not attend the party with his wife and son because he was crippled from an automobile accident the summer before and was confined to the house. Bebe Anna and Angeline Stokke had long been close friends, often visiting each other, sharing household duties, and entertaining together.

By Friday night, both women were feeling unusually fatigued, but they attributed their discomfort to overwork and indigestion. However, when Bebe Anna's son, Harry, died such a swift death on Saturday, the reality of their own condition became undeniable. By Saturday night, both Bebe Anna Chapiewski and Angeline Stokke lay on their deathbeds at the Chapiewski home, fully aware that the disease would claim them as well.

Angeline began showing symptoms of botulism sixteen hours after being poisoned by botulinum toxin. A detailed medical article in the Journal of the American Medical Association chronicled her case. In order of appearance, her symptoms were dizziness, muscular weakness, double vision, vomiting, constipation, difficulty swallowing, and muscular paralysis. Her respiration rate was normal, but very superficial and her pulse was 80 until the last hour when it became 120-140. Her temperature was normal and blood pressure was normal 125/75. Her physician described her condition as "marked quietude," and with no struggle. Angeline had extreme cyanosis causing her skin to turn blue from lack of oxygen. Just before she died, Angeline called her husband, Elmer, to her bedside and whispered to him in a hoarse voice, "I'm going to die." Reassuring words failed to change her conviction about her impending death. Elmer attempted to make her last moments easier. Angeline Stokke, age twenty-eight, died of respiratory collapse early on Sunday morning at 1:30 AM.

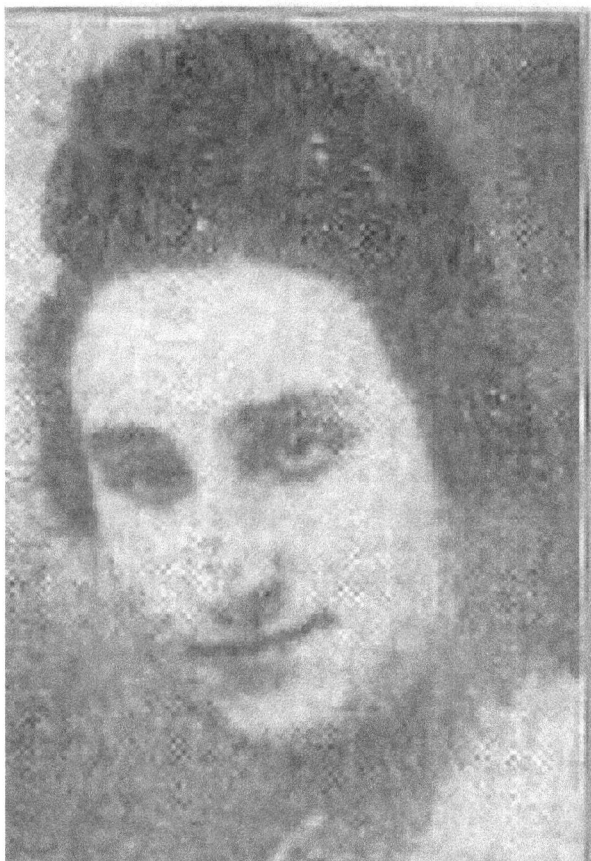

Angeline (Lessard) Stokke

Angeline Stokke and Bebe Chapiewski were friends to the end; they died within ten seconds of each other.

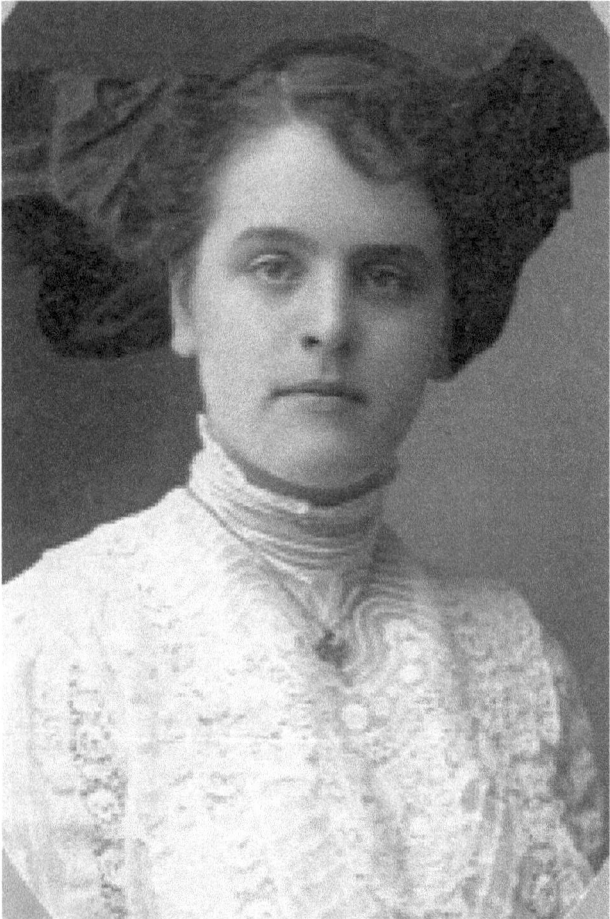

Bebe Anna (Greevers) Chapiewski

Earlier in the week, Elmer Stokke, Angeline's husband, had returned late Thursday evening from Fargo, where he had represented the Grafton

Chapter of the Royal Arch Masons at their annual convocation. Angeline had requested that Elmer "auto the whole group" (drive) to the Hein farm's late-night party, which he did. Upon their arrival, the hostess insisted Elmer try her homemade pea salad. Elmer politely declined, explaining that he wasn't hungry after his long trip. Elmer had a strict personal policy: he never ate vegetables. Refusing the salad was a decision that would save his life.

By Saturday, death was gripping the Hein household, too. There was no telephone in rural farm home so the Heins were unaware of the illnesses and deaths of their friends. The first to die was Delphine and Edward's eldest son, Edward J. Hein, Jr., age nineteen, who died at 7:30 AM on Saturday.

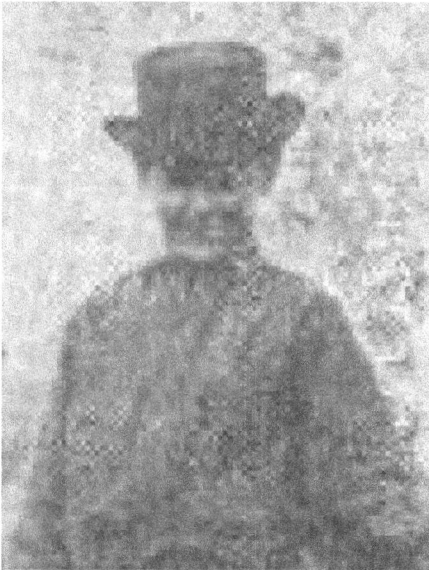

Edward J. Hein, Jr.

Next, the mother passed. Delphine LaFrombois Hein was the daughter of prominent Neche pioneers, the LaFrombois family, in Neche, North Dakota. Delphine Hein, age forty-six, died at 11:00 PM on Saturday, January 31.

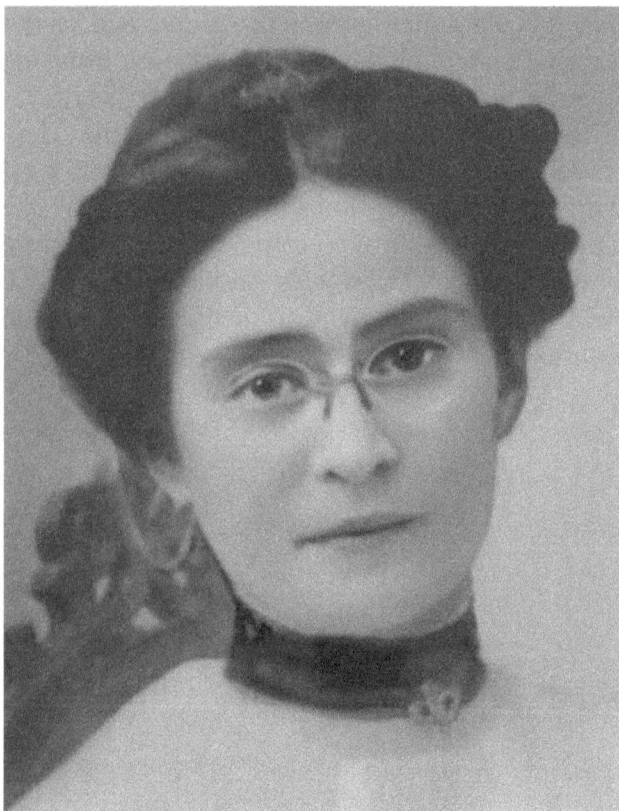

Delphine (LaFrombois) Hein

The eldest daughter, Elizabeth F. Hein, age twenty-one, died at 7:30 AM on Sunday.

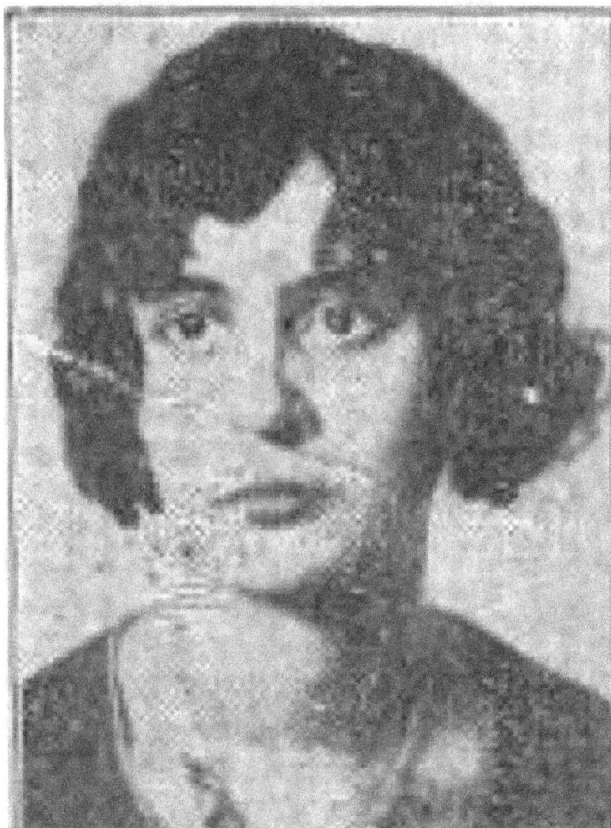

Elizabeth Hein

Edward Hein, Sr. spent his life farming. The last two years of his life he was in the dairy business and "was regarded as one of the most enterprising among the younger farmers." Edward Paul Hein, Sr., age forty-six, died at 10:30 PM on Sunday.

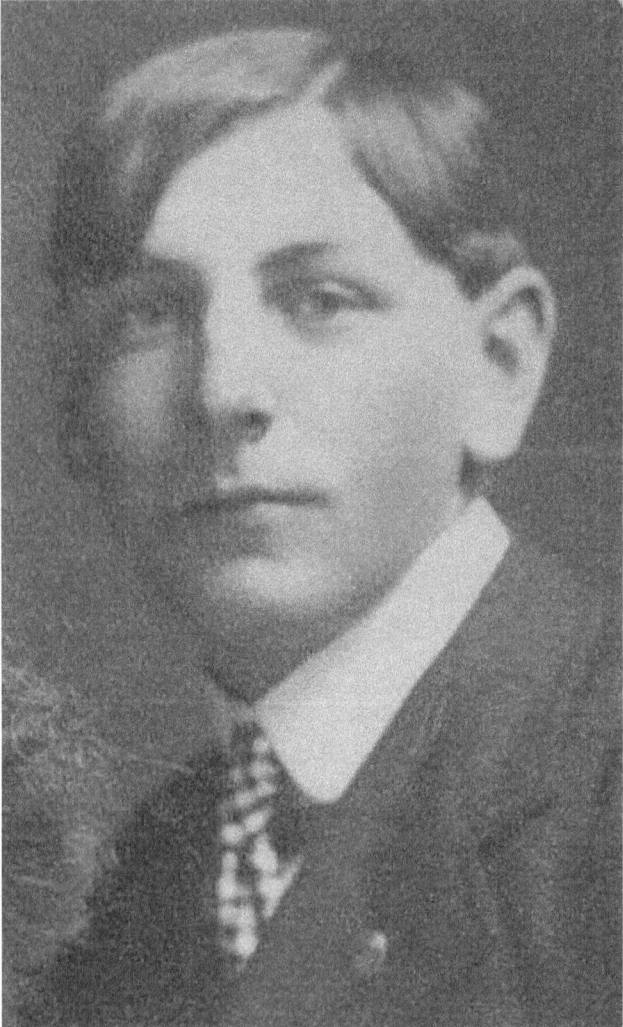

Edward Hein, Sr.

The last Hein to slip away was their youngest daughter, Genevieve Marie Hein, age sixteen, who died at 7:45 AM on Monday.

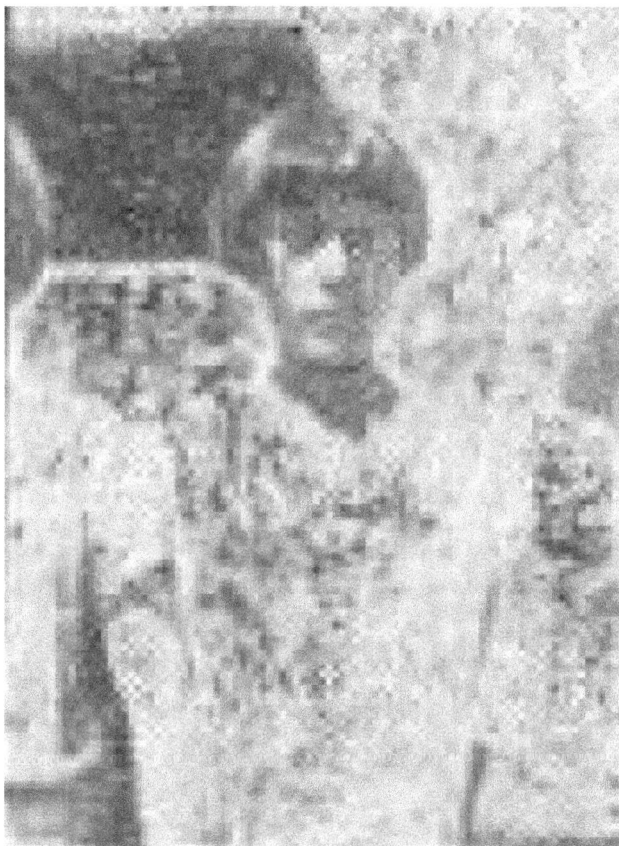

Genevieve Hein

Joseph Leach, a cousin of the Hein siblings, had come to live with his Aunt Delphine after the death of his mother in June 1921. In December of that same year, he married Irene Johnson. By 1925, Joseph was employed at DeSoto Creamery. A medical article chronicling the botulism outbreak later provided crucial details of Joseph's illness, shedding light on the complex nature of botulism left untreated by the antitoxin.

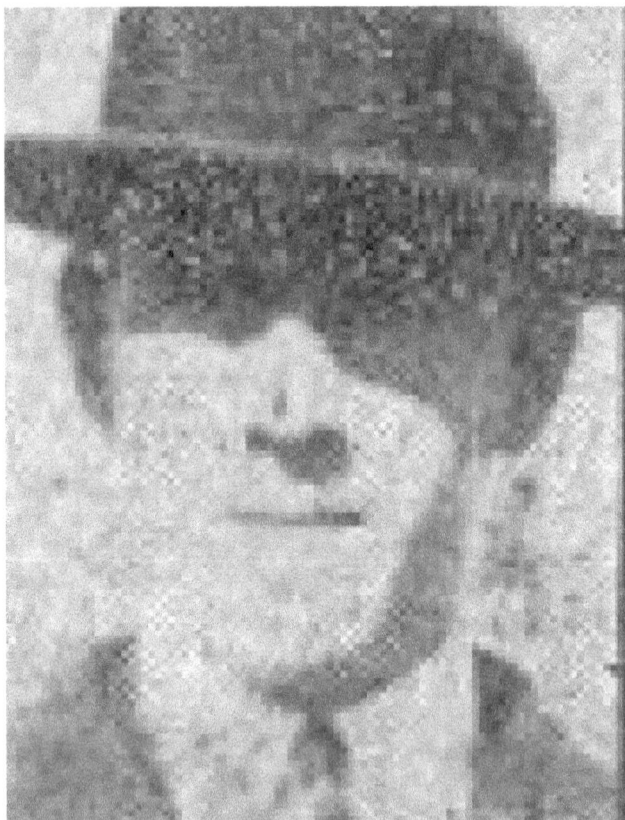

Joseph Leach

Joseph experienced symptoms thirty hours after ingesting the poison meal. On Saturday morning, he complained of dizziness, double vision, and nausea. Throughout the day, those symptoms persisted but did not worsen and no new symptoms appeared. On Sunday, he had diarrhea. He also had difficulty swallowing and talking; his tongue felt thick. His blood pressure was 115/70 and pulse 80 with a normal temperature. There was no muscle weakness until the second day of his symptoms. The first night he slept well, but the second night, he became restless. He experienced labored respiration.

Forty-eight hours after the symptoms began, the choking spells began, and he felt strangled in the throat frequently. This is when cyanosis developed as his skin turned bluish. His sensorium was clear to the end. Joseph Oliver Leach, age twenty-five, died at 12:00 PM on Monday in the hospital. The only autopsy of the outbreak was performed on him; the purpose was to confirm botulism as the cause of death. Joseph left behind a wife, and three children: Vivian Josephine, age four; Doris Ann, age three, and James Howard, an infant, age one month.

Arthur Lessard was hospitalized on Saturday. Although never in robust health, he was industrious and had been employed at the DeSoto Creamery and before that, with the Kiewel Cream Station. Arthur devoted most of his time to directing the Lessard orchestra. He was a cousin of Angeline Stokke. Arthur Lessard died in the hospital at 3:30 PM on Sunday.

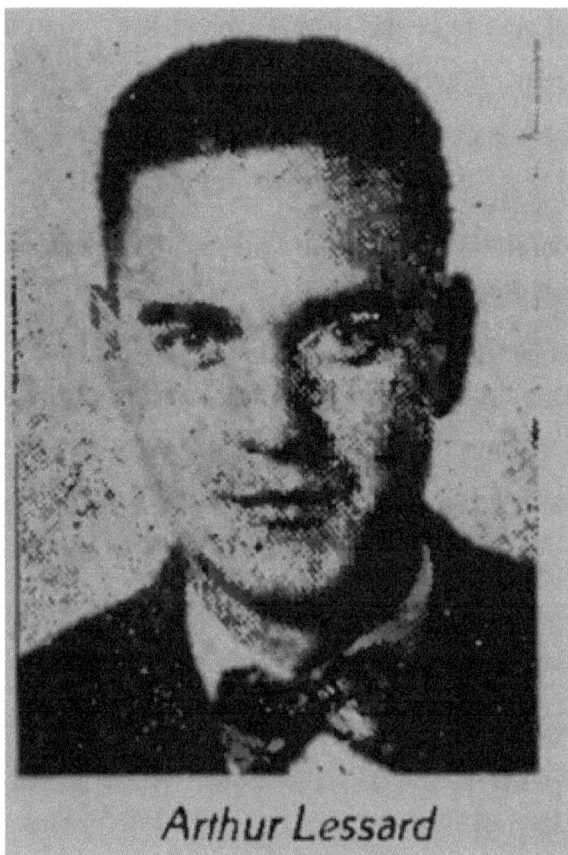

Arthur Lessard

Arthur Lessard

Marguerite McWilliams was also hospitalized on Saturday. She was a teacher at Grand Forks then moved to Grafton to work for the Northwestern Bell Telephone Company. Marguerite was the daughter of Mr. and Mrs. McWilliams of Bowesmont, North Dakota. She was in a hospital room down the hall from Arthur Lessard. Marguerite McWilliams died in the hospital at 3:30 PM on Sunday.

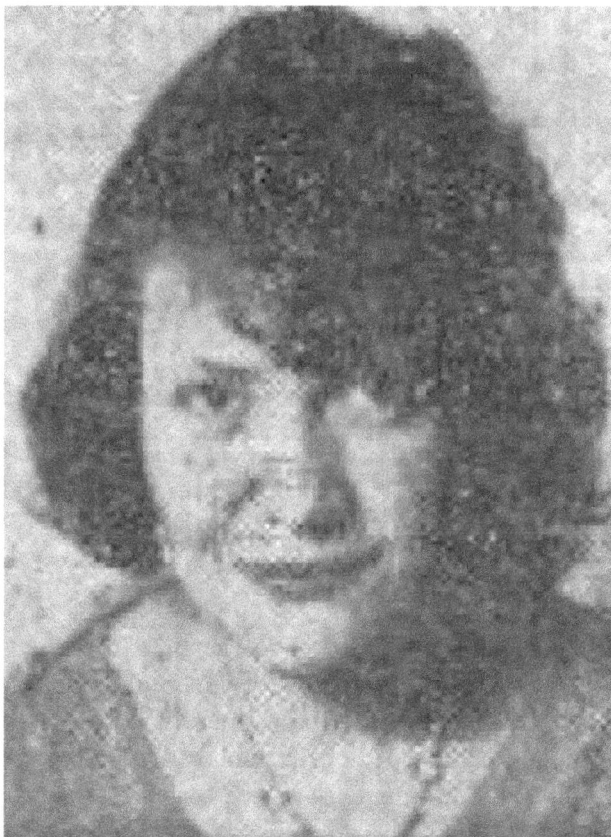

Marguerite McWilliams

The thirteenth and final victim was Winfield A. Ware, a young man whose death marked the tragic end of the outbreak. A 1927 graduate of Grafton High School, Winfield was known for his athleticism, playing on the school's football team. After graduation, he enlisted in the North Dakota National Guard. Throughout his brief life, Winfield held various jobs, including work for H.G. Sprague, a pioneering grocer and potato buyer in the area. His untimely death was the last in a string of fatalities that rocked the Grafton community.

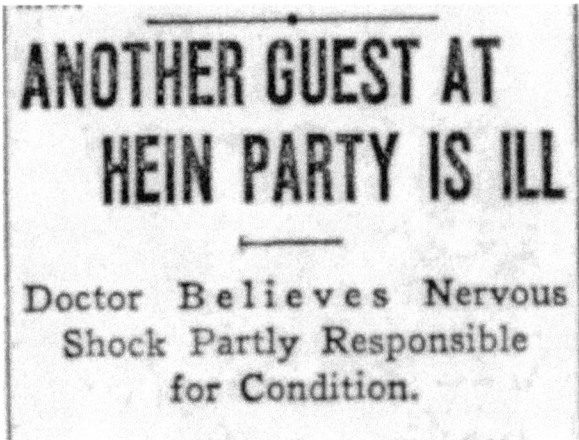

ANOTHER GUEST AT HEIN PARTY IS ILL

Doctor Believes Nervous Shock Partly Responsible for Condition.

Winfield had carefully removed the peas from his vegetable salad, yet he was still struck by a delayed case of botulism. Despite avoiding the direct consumption of the contaminated food, he ultimately suffered the same fatal outcome as his friends—though his death came ten days after the party. The *Grafton News & Times* chronicled the unusual case of Winfield:

"Following the fatal participation in the botulinus-infested salad lunch served at midnight, January 29, Winfield Ware had a slight attack of nausea and was apparently relieved.

Was Well Sunday and Monday: Friday and Saturday following he was well and Sunday evening he assisted C.L. Schumacher and his father, both Masonic secretaries in preparing circular matter for mailing. Nothing was amiss Monday.

Was Weak Tuesday: Tuesday he responded to a fire alarm, fell and was assisted to his feet by Jack Munroe, and complained of weakness and affected vision. This was his last day about town and spent the rest of the week with his father.

Attended Inquest Wednesday: Although weak, he was able to attend the coroner's inquest Wednesday, but his condition did not excite the serious apprehension of his physician. At the coroner's inquest, he testified that he ate only a very small portion of the salad and had not, as he remembered, eaten any of the peas which were at first believed to have harbored the deadly poison. Much of his trouble was attributed to nervousness.

Witnessed Hein Funeral Friday: Friday he sat at the window and witnessed the heart-rending funeral of the Edward Hein family and Joseph Leach, as the bodies of his six companions were accorded the solace and blessing of the Church.

<u>To Hospital Friday Evening</u>: Friday evening Dr. C. J. Glaspel, who attended him, ordered him taken to the Grafton Deaconess Hospital and visitors were excluded from his room. Although not considered dangerously ill, he had developed positive symptoms of botulism. His vision was poor and difficulty in swallowing was experienced. No marked change in his condition was apparent Saturday, and when visited by his father that evening was cheerful and complained of no particular pain.

<u>Died Sunday Morning</u>: About 6 o'clock Sunday morning a change for the worse was evident and his father was summoned. He was able to enjoy a bowl of soup and a glass of milk which were given him at 7:30, and less than 20 minutes later, while resting after this light repast, his life ceased its worldly pilgrimage and he was summoned hence as the 13th victim of the greatest tragedy that has ever darkened this community."

Several key observations emerge from this newspaper account. Winfield and his physicians initially underestimated the severity of his condition due to the delayed onset of symptoms. Despite witnessing the deaths of twelve of his friends, both he and his doctors believed he would recover from what appeared to be a mild case of botulism.

Winfield's symptoms developed slowly and seemed less severe compared to the others. Additionally, health officials investigating the outbreak dismissed his concerns, attributing his symptoms to nervousness rather than recognizing the threat of botulism. Understandably, Winfield had not eaten much food since the party, and doctors thought that accounted for his weakened condition. Dr. Allen, a member of the coroner's inquiry, reported that Winfield Ware was "regarded in Grafton as a very unreliable party" and added that his nickname was "Windy Ware." The term windy implies a person is known for empty, prolonged, boastful talk with the goal of impressing others. This negative bias regarding Winfield's personality contributed to the tragic delay in addressing the status of his health, which ultimately led to his death.

WINFIELD WARE, 23, DIES 9 DAYS AFTER LUNCH IN GRAFTON HOME

'Only Tasted' Of Deadly, Salad, Latest Victim Said At Inquest

WENT TO HOSPITAL ON FRIDAY NIGHT

Illness First Thought Nervous Reaction Of Experience

Dr. William Carey from the University of Chicago delivered the botulism antitoxin, which had been supplied by the only commercially available source at the time: Jensen and Salisbury, Inc. of Kansas City, Missouri. Although the antitoxin was available to treat Winfield, it was not administered because his case did not initially appear life-threatening. His symptoms, developing slowly and seeming less severe than those of the other victims, led medical professionals to mistakenly believe that Winfield would recover without the antitoxin. The *Fargo Forum* newspaper reported that Winfield's pulse "mounted rapidly to 145 beats" during his last hours of life. He also ran a temperature of 101-102 degrees for two days prior to the end. Winfield Ware, who would have turned twenty-three the next month, died of mild botulism at 7:40 AM on Sunday, February 8. He was buried next to his mother who had died when Winfield was thirteen years old.

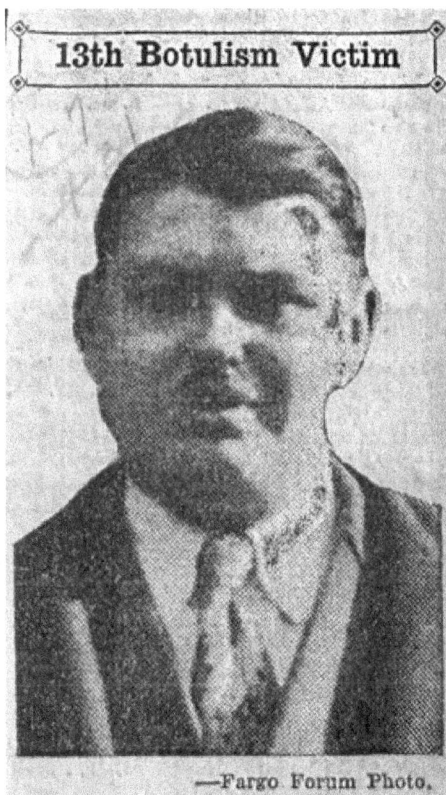

13th Botulism Victim

—Fargo Forum Photo.

Winfield Ware

After Winfield Ware died, the doctors felt it was imperative to treat the others who attended the party yet showed no symptoms: Helen Seick, Moses Lessard, and his girlfriend Ellen Burke, age sixteen, who was a waitress at the Grafton Cafe. Helen Seick worked as a beauty shop operator in Grafton, but after the tragedy, she had gone back to her parent's home in Moorhead, Minnesota. Dr. W.H. Long, who administered the antitoxin to Helen, reported that she had been very ill and her legs were weak. She had also fainted when attempting to climb the stairs to retire to bed. She had nystagmus (rapid involuntary eye movements) until the fourth day and she also developed a mild serum reaction. Her physician reported that she completely recovered, but did not specify to what degree or how long recovery took. Moses and Ellen declined the antitoxin treatment—and remarkably, they survived. They were married six months later.

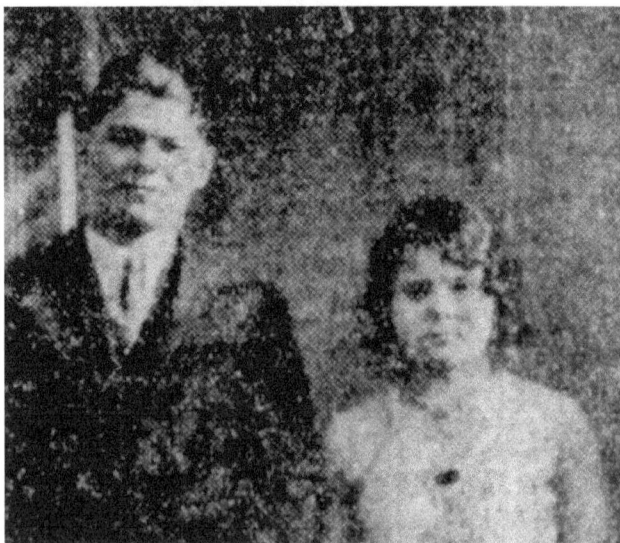

Moses Lessard and Ellen Burke

The entire community of Grafton was grief-stricken, but none more so than the three surviving Hein boys. The *Grand Forks Herald* described the tragic scene to its readers:

"Three little boys cried themselves to sleep here tonight, wondering at the strange fate that had taken from them their father, mothers, two sisters, and their big brother. In strange beds at the homes of relatives here, the three young survivors of the Ed Hein family found little solace in the efforts to comfort them. It was "Daddy" and "Mother" they wanted. Richard, 14 years old, Wilfred, 12, and Marvin, 4, escaped the menace of the poisoned food that took lives at the Hein home Thursday night only because they were "too young" to stay up so late. Out at the Hein farm, two miles north of Grafton, a little black and white dog wondered, too, at the strange fate that had taken away his young masters. Forlornly he sat at the side of the little yellow house, patiently waiting the homecoming of friends."

The oldest son was quoted in the *Walsh County Record* as stating, "Please will you see that our mother's wedding ring is saved so that we have something to remember her by."

By 1931, medical literature on botulism was both extensive and informative, with laboratory tests available to detect botulinum toxin in food, stool, and serum. Most physicians had developed reliable diagnostic skills based on clinical symptoms alone. None of the four physicians treating the victims in the Grafton outbreak had ever encountered a case of botulism in person. Yet, despite their lack of direct experience, they were able to diagnose the illness with confidence before the first victim had even died.

Dr. Robert Allen, the state epidemiologist, co-authored a medical paper with A. Walter Ecklund, M.S., a bacteriologist. They published their case report on the North Dakota botulism outbreak in the Journal of the American Medical Association. In the article they stated,

"The diagnosis of botulism, although a rare disease, from the clinical symptoms alone, when established entails no serious entanglements to the trained mind of the skilled physician."

This single sentence encapsulates a critical issue that has persisted in nearly every botulism case and outbreak over the years: diagnosing botulism requires a physician's ability to recognize its symptoms, even though the disease is rare and often the presentations include atypical symptoms.

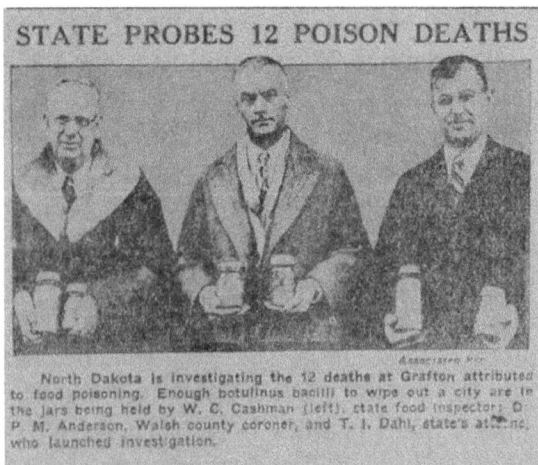

STATE PROBES 12 POISON DEATHS

North Dakota is investigating the 12 deaths at Grafton attributed to food poisoning. Enough botulinus bacilli to wipe out a city are in the jars being held by W. C. Cashman (left), state food inspector; D P. M. Anderson, Walsh county coroner, and T. I. Dahl, state's attorney, who launched investigation.

W.C. Cashman, P.M. Anderson, T.I. Dahl holding canning specimens from the Hein cellar.

TAKEAWAYS from
THE NORTH DAKOTA OUTBREAK

There is variability in the symptoms even within the same botulism outbreak.

Botulism symptoms wax and wane which gives hope for recovery, only to suddenly result in a fatal outcome.

Botulism patients often underestimate their condition's severity; sudden decline and death can surprise both patient and physician.

Botulism symptoms unfold at a different pace for each patient and can also present with different severities for each patient. Even when all cases experience fatal outcomes, the progression varies greatly.

Death can occur two weeks after ingestion of poison. as numerous animal models testing for toxicity have shown for decades,
the lower the dose, the longer the time to death.

Exercise can strain the diaphragm muscles and cause breathing difficulties.

Complete respiratory collapse from botulism can happen with little to no warning, resulting in death within minutes.

ABOUT THE AUTHOR

J.A. Talkington, PhD, is a professor and researcher in the field of entrepreneurship and innovation, driven by a deep curiosity that led to an unexpected passion for the history of botulism. This unique pursuit of this obscure subject led to revive a nearly forgotten perspective, that of a botulism historian.

Inspired by the 1920s archival collection at Stanford University, the resulting research became *Recognizing Botulism*–a complete reinvention of how physicians and patients today can use a century-old approach to understand the complex constellation of symptoms that are characteristic of botulism. The purpose of this book was to assemble a medical narrative about botulism that included the atypical symptoms so as to complete the clinical picture.

The hope is that anyone who reads these 120 cases reviewed in this book will develop new insights that are useful to recognize botulism.

ABOUT THE RESEARCH:
PAST AND FUTURE

The Far Past

Each era of botulism research carries its own unique voice and character. When you trace the timeline from 1890 to 1980, you can almost feel the shifting tides—curiosity intertwined with ignorance, moments of wonder shadowed by revelations of horror, and bursts of confidence tempered by desperation. The only consistent quality to every era was the feeling of helplessness the physicians expressed when they realized they faced a case of botulism. In this research, you encounter a mix of public duty, corporate malfeasance, ethical violations, courageous stands for integrity, and an unwavering devotion to the pursuit of knowledge. In many ways, not much has changed. The cycles repeat, with history echoing through each new generation of researchers. The world, it seems, is a stage, and it falls to the researcher to discern the bad actors from the good ones, identifying which voices deserve trust and which are suspect.

One particularly captivating person from Stanford University in the 1920s was Georgina Brackenridge Spooner Burke. A pioneer among females in the sciences, Georgina was married to a man with a PhD in microbiology, but she held her own master's degree and carved out her own path in the world of scientific research.

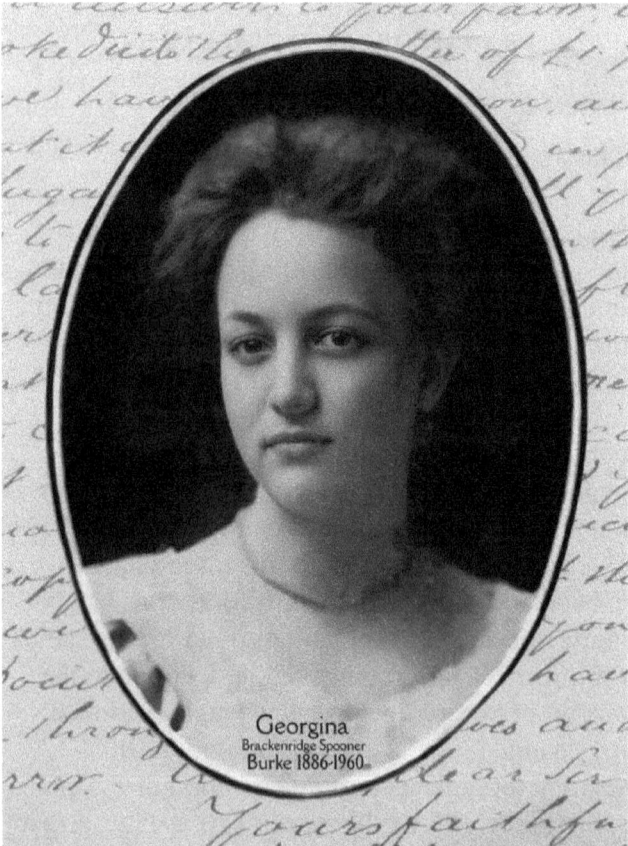

Georgina Brackenridge Spooner at Vassar, 1907

She had spent years in the Laboratory of Bacteriology and Experimental Pathology researching alongside of Dr. Dickson. Her papers such as "*A Study of the Resistance of the Spores of Bacillus Botulinus to Various Sterilizing Agencies which are Commonly Employed in the Canning of Fruits and Vegetables* made her the rare expert on the conditions necessary to prevent the production of botulinum toxin in canned foods.

In a bold move, Georgina publicly challenged Dr. Milton Joseph Rosenau, Professor of Preventive Medicine and Hygiene of the Harvard Medical School accusing him—and by extension, his institution—of a serious ethical breach. In a national publication, she claimed that Harvard's findings on the safety of commercially canned foods were compromised by a financial conflict of interest, as the research had been funded by a $225,000 grant from the National Canners Association and the California Canners League. According to Georgina, these industry ties skewed the results, as the Harvard study had concluded that botulism was only a risk in home-canned goods, not commercially processed foods. Georgina's lab tests showed the toxin production occurred in both sources of canned food. At great peril to her career Georgina spoke up, knowing that Harvard's misrepresentation of the risks would cost lives. Her accusation was not only audacious but valid, and it shed light on a troubling pattern: in academia–research funded by corporate interests sometimes comes with an agenda. Sadly, such conflicts of interest continue to shape research in higher education today, where corporate dollars can sometimes drive conclusions more than scientific integrity.

The Recent Past

I can count on one hand the number of studies on long-term recovery from botulism that have been published in the past 130 years. For long-term outcomes about the botulism survivors discussed in *Recognizing Botulism*, I had to dig through obituaries and old newspaper articles from 1902 to 1960 to find any mention of their names or health status. Many times, I discovered irrelevant factoids such as that most of the Pi Beta Phi members at Stanford University who survived the botulism outbreak in 1913 were married shortly after graduation. In fact, the Class of 1914 boasted one of the highest marriage rates in the history of the university at the time. The fact they tracked that data amazes me.

I also managed to track down Dr. J.A.R. Glancy's grandson to ask about his grandfather's longevity and cause of death after surviving the botulism outbreak in the Yukon Territory in 1919. My apologies to every Glancy in Canada whom I emailed during that search; I was desperately trying to find any clues about the doctor's health in his later years. What turned out to be more useful, however, was information about survivors' quality of life after recovering from the acute phase of botulism. A small breakthrough came when I found a child involved in the 1919 Ohio outbreak who, in his later years, shared an oral history of the event that was archived by the local library in the 1980s. He recalled that his mother's eyesight was never quite as sharp after recovering from botulism.

These findings—scattered, anecdotal fragments—are at best "research crumbs." But they have provided invaluable glimpses into the long-term effects of botulism, a topic that remains underexplored in the scientific literature.

Most botulism case reports published in academic journals end with a simple line: "The patient recovered and was discharged after XX days." Some papers go even further, stating, "This case was completely resolved," which is highly unlikely. In my own interviews with individuals who survived botulism and were treated with the antitoxin, some forty years after their initial episodes, it is clear that the effects of the disease often persist for decades. Relapse episodes are so common that patients themselves have coined terms like "toxy" or "botchy" to describe those episodic flare-ups from botulism damage.

For many recovering from botulism, the search for information on long-term outcomes and healing protocols is fraught with frustration. They crave hope and guidance, but reliable, evidence-based information is scant. What remains are reports only on severe botulism (not mild), anecdotal evidence, and an overwhelming sense of uncertainty about the road to full recovery.

The Future

I have developed and vetted a comprehensive survey tool specifically designed to document and track patients' recoveries from botulism. The goal is to use this tool in longitudinal studies that will follow patients over time. This initiative is a critical step toward filling the gaps in botulism research and improving outcomes for those affected by this debilitating condition.

Contact Information

J.A. Talkington, PhD

Email: RecognizingBotulism@gmail.com
Facebook: RecognizingBotulism
Instagram: Recognizing_Botulism
YouTube: @recognizingbotulism

References

Preface

McDonough, Stephen L. *The Golden Ounce: a Century of Public Health in North Dakota.* University Printing Center, 1989.

ST Louis, Michael E., et al. "Botulism from chopped garlic: delayed recognition of a major outbreak." *Annals of Internal Medicine* 108.3 (1988): 363-368.

Zeide, Anna. "The Botulism Outbreak That Gave Rise to America's Food Safety System." 2018. https://www.smithsonianmag.com /history/botulism-outbreak-gave-rise-americas-food-safety-system-180969868/

There are only two technical books on botulism: *Botulism: A Clinical and Experimental Study* by Ernest Dickson, MD, of Stanford University (1918).

Botulism: The Organism, its Toxins, the Disease by Louis D.S. Smith, PhD (1977).

Each case of botulism is legally required to be reported to the state health department, which then notifies the Centers for Disease Control and Prevention (CDC) in Atlanta, Georgia. (The 24/7 botulism line at the CDC is (770) 488-7100.) The CDC holds the botulism antitoxin and evaluates whether the severity justifies releasing the antitoxin to the patient with botulism.

Chapter 1

The Beach and Cliff House, San Francisco –
1902. Library of Congress, Prints and
Photographs Division, Washington,
LC-USZ6-1371 (b & w film copy
neg.).

Jellinek, E. O. "Ptomaine Poisoning."
California State Journal of Medicine,
vol. 1, no. 4, 1903, p. 121.
A free PDF download from NIH found
through Google Scholar.

Lamanna, Carl. "The Most Poisonous Poison:
What Do We Know About the Toxin of
Botulism? What Are the Problems to Be
Solved?" *Science*, vol. 130, no. 3378,
1959, pp. 763-772.

San Francisco Call and Post. 4 Dec. 1902, p. 4;
14 Dec. 1902, p. 45.

San Francisco Chronicle. 14 Dec. 1902, p.
15.

Notable Interest:
The boarding house is still standing
and is located on the northwest corner
of Divisadero and McAllister. The
building currently accommodates two
restaurants.

Chapter 2

Black, S. "Pathology of Ptomaine
    Poisoning." *Southern California
    Practitioner*, vol. 22, 1907.

Carter, Henry, and Mabel Carter. *The Los
    Angeles Times*, 5 Jan. 1907.
    Cucamonga Canyon Map, 1910. PastMaps,
    https://pastmaps.com/explore/us/ca/san-
    bernardino/rancho-cucamonga

Group of Citrus Groves in Southern
    California. ca. 1900, California
    Historical Society Collection,
    University of Southern California.

Hutson, Cliff. Cucamonga Peak. Later cropped
    and color-edited by Daniel Case,
    Wikimedia Commons, CC BY 2.0,
    https://commons.wikimedia.org/
    w/index.php?curid=3407272

Morrow, Glenn, and Tracy. Grave Marker of
    Charles Abbott. Find a Grave,
    10285281/charles-edward-abbott

The Los Angeles Times. 5 Jan. 1907, p. 13.

Oakland Tribune. 12 July 1908, p. 27

The Pomona Daily Review. Pomona, California,
    5 1907.

The Register. Santa Ana, California, 8 Jan.
    1907, p. 3.

The San Bernardino County Sun. San
Bernardino, California, 4 Jan. 1907, p. 4; 5
Jan 1907 p.1.

The San Bernardino County Sun. 4 Jan.
1907.

The San Francisco Call and Post. San
Francisco, California, 5 Jan. 1907, p. 2.

Chapter 3

The Daily Nonpareil. Council Bluffs, Iowa, 14 Dec. 1913, p. 11.

The Des Moines Register. Des Moines, Iowa, 15 Dec. 1913, p. 10.

Dickson, E. C. Botulism: A Clinical and Experimental Study. 1918.
Free download at Google Books.
https://www.ncbi.nlm.nih.gov/pmc/articles/PMC2128451/pdf/327.pdf

"Ray Lyman Wilbur Family Photo." Wikimedia Commons, uploaded by MohenjoDaro, CC BY-SA 3.0,
https://commons.wikimedia.org/w/index.php?curid=8354021.

The Register. Santa Ana, California, 9 Dec. 1913, p. 1.

Oakland Tribune. Oakland, California, 9 Dec. 1913, p. 1; 9 Dec. 1913, p. 7; 12 Dec. 1913, p. 7.

San Bernardino News and The Free Press. San Bernardino, California, 9 Dec. 1913, p. 1.

The San Francisco Call and Post. San Francisco, California, 9 Dec. 1913, p. 1; 10 Dec. 1913, p. 8.

San Francisco Chronicle. San Francisco, California, 12 Dec. 1913, p. 4.

Wilbur, Ray Lyman, and William Ophüls. "Botulism: A Report of Food-Poisoning Apparently Due to Eating of Canned String Beans, with Pathological Report of a Fatal Case." *Archives of Internal Medicine*, vol. 14, no. 4, 1914, pp. 589-604. Free PDF download on Google Scholar.

Woodland Daily Democrat. Woodland, California, 11 Dec. 1913, p. 1; 12 Dec 1913, p. 1; 12 Dec. 1913, p. 1.

Chapter 4

"Action Cardiaque Propriétés Spécialité de
la Botuline." *Biologie, Comptes
Rendus*, 10th ser., 1897.

The Alturas New Era. Alturas, California,
Friday, 26 Sept. 1919, p. 1.

California State Board of Health. *California
State Board of Health Report*, vol. 15,
no. 4, 1919, p. 114.

The Colusa Daily Sun. Colusa, California,
23 Sept. 1919, p. 1; 24 Sept. 1919,
p. 1; 27 Sept. 1919, p. 4; 26
Sept. 1919; 3 Oct. 1919; 4 Oct.
1919; 31 Dec. 1919, p. 1.

Colusa Sun-Herald. Colusa, California,
31 July 1919, p. 4, 11 Sept. 1919, p. 4;
20 Sept. 1919, p. 1; 23 Sept. 1919, p. 1;
2 Oct. 1919, p. 1, Oct. 1919, p. 1; 9 Oct.
1919, p. 1; 31 Dec 1919, p. 1.

Kelly, Frank. "Investigation of Five Cases of
Botulinus Poisoning at Colusa September
30, 1919." *County California State Board
of Health Report*, vol. 15, no. 4, 1919, p.
114.

O'Leary, Peter. Family Portrait at the Estate.
O'Leary Family Estate, 1920.

The Sacramento Bee. Sacramento, California, Fri., 26 Sept. 1919, p. 5; 1 Oct. 1919, p. 8; Mon., 6 Oct. 1919, p. 9.

Tacket, Carol O., et al. "Equine Antitoxin Use and Other Factors That Predict Outcome in type A Foodborne Botulism." *The American Journal of Medicine*, vol. 76, no. 5, 1984, pp. 794-798.

Willows Daily Journal. Willows, California, Thu., 25 Sept. 1919, p. 1; Tue., 23 Sept. 1919, p. 1; Sat., 4 Oct. 1919, p. 1.

Notable Interest:

Cash Martin's daughter also became a newspaper writer for The Willows Daily newspaper when she was 18 using the byline of "Miss Goldie Martin." She was just 4 when her father died.

Chapter 5

Bresee, Randall R. Dawson Cemetery. RandallRBreseePhoto.com, www.RandallRBreseePhoto.com.

The Edmonton Bulletin. Mon., 9 June 1919, p. 12.

Dawson Daily News. Dawson, Yukon, Canada, Mon., 18 Aug. 1919, p. 4.

Dawson Historical Society. Personal communication, August 2024.

Glancy, James Albert Ray. "Botulism—A Clinical Study of an Outbreak in the Yukon." *Canadian Medical Association Journal*, vol. 10, no. 11, 1920, p. 1027.
Free PDF download from the National Institutes of Health, National Library of Medicine.

The Hamilton Spectator. Hamilton, Ontario, Canada, 4 June 1919, p. 13.

The Leader-Post. Regina, Saskatchewan, Canada, Wed., 4 June 1919, p. 1.

Lincoln Journal Star. Lincoln, Nebraska, 4 June 1919, p. 3.

The Ottawa Herald. Ottawa, Kansas, 4
   June 1919, p. 6.

Reading Times. Reading, Pennsylvania, 5
   June 1919, p. 4.

Reno Gazette-Journal. Reno, Nevada, Wed.,
   28 May 1919, p. 1.

The Seattle Star. Seattle, Washington, 4 June
   1919, p. 4.

Star Weekly. Toronto, Ontario, Canada, Sat., 26
   Feb. 1921, p. 10.

Tonopah Daily Bonanza. Tonopah, Nevada,
   Fri., 6 June 1919, p. 4.

Whitehorse Daily Star. Whitehorse, Yukon,
   Canada, Fri., 12 Jan. 1917, p. 4; Fri.,
   30 May 1919, p. 1; Fri., 22 Aug. 1919,
   p 4.

The Evening Review. 28 Aug. 1919, pp. 1,
   4; 27 June 1919, p. 4; 19 Sept. 1919, p.
   1; 14 Nov. 1919, p. 3.

Chapter 6

The Akron Beacon Journal. Akron, Ohio, 27
    Aug. 1919, p. 1; 28 Sep 28, p. 1; 27 S
    Sep 27, 1919, p. 9; 2 Sep. 1919, p.15;
    15 Sep 1919, p.3.

The Alliance Review and Leader. Alliance,
    Ohio, 8 Aug. 1919.

Armstrong, Charles. "Botulism from Eating
    Canned Ripe Olives." *Journal of
    Medical Research*, 1919.
    Free PDF download on Google Scholar

Battle Creek Enquirer. Battle Creek,
    Michigan, 26 Aug. 1919, p. 1; 27 Sep,
    1919, p.1.

The Bucyrus Evening Telegraph. Bucyrus,
    Ohio, 4 Nov. 1919, p. 1.

The Cincinnati Enquirer. Cincinnati, Ohio,
    27 Aug. 1919, p. 3; 5 Sep. 1919, p. 9.

The Coshocton Tribune. Coshocton, Ohio,
    26 Aug. 1919, p. 8.

The Daily Times. New Philadelphia, Ohio,
    26 Aug. 1919, p. 1.

The Dayton Herald. Dayton, Ohio, 27 Aug.
    1919, p. 1.

The Evening Review. East Liverpool, Ohio, 27, 1919, p. 1; 28 Aug. 1919, p. 1. Fort Scott Daily Tribune and Fort Scott Daily Monitor. Fort Scott, Kansas, 28 Feb. 1918, p. 7.

Lakeside Country Club, Canton, Ohio. Digital Collections, Miami University, https://digital.lib.miamioh.edu/ digital/collection/postcards/id/5251.

The Marion Star. Marion, Ohio, 30 Aug. 1919, p. 2.

Morgan, Williams H., Jr. Ohio History Connection, Alliance Public Library, 1980. www.ohiomemory.org/digital/collection /p16007coll36/id/9288

The Ohio Laborer. Licking, Ohio, 28 Aug. 1919, p. 1.

The Salem News. Salem, Ohio, 20 Dec. 1949, p. 1.

The Sandusky Register. Sandusky, Ohio, 27 Aug. 1919, p. 1.

The Times Recorder. Zanesville, Ohio, 27 Aug. 1919, p. 2; 28 Aug. 1919, p. 1.

The Tribune. Coshocton, Ohio, 27 Aug. 1919, p. 1.

The Zanesville Signal. Zanesville, Ohio, 30
      Aug. 1919, p. 1.

Notable Interest:
      Two years after this botulism outbreak
      in Alliance, Dr. Phillips would become
      one of the four founding physicians
      who established The Cleveland Clinic,
      a hospital that became known for
      medical research.

Chapter 7

Bisbee Daily Review. Bisbee, Arizona, 5
Nov. 1919, p. 2.

Daily Arkansas Gazette. 29 Feb. 1920, p. 76.

Detroit Free Press. Detroit, Michigan, 24
Oct. 1919, p. 1; 25 Oct. 1919, p. 1; 26
Oct. 1919, p. 1; 26 Oct. 1919, p. 3; 27
Oct. 1919, p. 6; 28 Oct. 1919, p. 1; 30
Oct. 1919, p. 1; 20 Jan. 1920, p. 1; 13
Feb. 1921, p. 1; 28 Oct. 1928, p. 12; 5
Jan. 1920 p. 98; 15 Nov. 1944, p. 16;
26 Jul. 1950, p. 12; 28 Jan. 1951, p. 7;
25 April 1919, p. 5; 30 Jun. 1963, p.
118.

Jennings, C. G., et al. "An Outbreak of
Botulism: Report of Cases." *Journal of
the American Medical Association*,
vol. 74, no. 2, 1920, pp. 77-80.

Lansing State Journal. Lansing, Michigan,
16 Nov. 1945, p. 26.

The News Scimitar. 7 Feb. 1920, p. 1.

The Philadelphia Inquirer. Philadelphia,
Pennsylvania, 30 Nov. 1919, p. 74.

Notable Interest:
The history of the Sales' 1918 mansion
"Edgeroad"
https://www.higbiemaxon.com

/blog/historical-architecture-of-grosse-pointe-251-lincoln-road.html
About the architect, Louis Kamper. https://historicdetroit.org /architects/louis-kamper
According to Zillow, Edgeroad sold in 2022 for $2,900,000 as 251 Lincoln Rd, Grosse Pointe, MI 48230. www.zillow.com/homedetails/ 251-Lincoln-Rd-Grosse-Pointe-MI-48230/88253342_zpid/. Accessed 28 Nov. 2024.

Chapter 8

Detroit Free Press, 20 Jan. 1920, p. 1.

Fort Scott Daily Tribune and Fort Scott Daily Monitor. 17 Jan. 1920, p. 1.

Hot Springs New Era. 17 Jan. 1920, p. 4; 18 Jan. 1920, p. 6.

Middletown Times Herald. 16 Jan. 1920, p. 4.

Moberly Democrat. 18 Jan. 1920, p. 1.

New York Daily Herald. 19 Jan. 1920, p. 3.

The New York Times. 18 Jan. 1920, p. 9.

New-York Tribune. 18 Jan. 1920, p. 15; 19 Jan. 1920, p. 6.

The Ogden Standard-Examiner. 17 Jan. 1920, p. 1.

Sisco, Dwight L. "An Outbreak of Botulism." *Journal of the American Medical Association* 74.8 (1920): 516-521.

Young, James Harvey. "Botulism and the ripe olive scare of 1919-1920." *Bulletin of the History of Medicine* 50.3 (1976): 372-391.

Chapter 9

Asbury Park Press. Asbury Park, New Jersey, 5
Feb. 1920, p. 4. The Commercial Appeal.
Memphis, Tennessee, 8 Feb. 1920; 11 Feb.
1920.

Emerson, Herbert W., and George W. Collins.
"Botulism from Canned Ripe Olives."
*Journal of Laboratory and Clinical
Medicine*, vol. 5, 1920, pp. 559-565.

The News Scimitar. Memphis, Tennessee, 7 Feb.
1920, p. 1; 10 Feb. 1920, p. 1; 11 Feb.
1920.

Chapter 10

Geiger, J. C. "An Outbreak of Botulism at St. Anthony's Hospital, Oakland, Calif., October, 1920." *Public Health Reports*, 1920, pp. 2858-2860.

Martinez Daily Standard. Martinez, California, 22 Oct. 1920, p. 4.

San Francisco Chronicle. San Francisco, California, 21 Oct. 1920, p. 2.

Oakland Enquirer. Oakland, California, 20 Oct. 1920, p. 1.

Oakland Tribune. Oakland, California, 20 Oct. 1920, p. 1.

Chapter 11

Emerson, Herbert W., and George W. Collins.
"Botulism from Canned Ripe Olives."
Journal of Laboratory and Clinical Medicine, vol. 5, 1920, pp. 559-565.

The Journal of the American Medical Association, vol. 74, Jan.-Mar. 1920.

The Long Beach Telegram. Long Beach, California, 25 Feb. 1921, p. 7

The News Scimitar. Memphis, Tennessee, 7 Feb. 1920, p. 1; 9 Feb. 1920, p. 1.

Oakland Tribune. Oakland, California, 20 Oct. 1920, p. 1.

The Commercial Appeal. Memphis, Tennessee, 8 Feb. 1920; 11 Feb. 1920.

Chapter 12

Albany Democrat. Albany, Oregon, 4 Feb. 1924,
    p. 1; 14 Feb. 1924, p. 2; 14 Feb.
    1924, p. 2; 21 Feb. 1924, p. 5; 14
    Feb. 1924, p. 2.

Albany Daily Democrat. Albany, Oregon, 4 Feb.
    1924, p. 1; 7 Feb. 1924, p. 1; 11
    Feb. 1924, p. 4; 13 Feb. 1924, p. 1.

Lincoln Journal Star. Lincoln, Nebraska, 31 Mar.
    1924, p. 8.

The San Francisco Examiner. San Francisco,
    California, 5 Feb. 1924, p. 1.

Star Tribune. Minneapolis, Minnesota, 23 Mar.
    1924, p. 73.

Photo credit: *The Times-News*. Twin Falls, Idaho,
    21 Feb. 1924, p. 2.

Stricker, Frederick D., and Jacob Casson Geiger.
    "Outbreaks of Botulism at Albany,
    Oregon, and Sterling, Colorado,
    February, 1924." *Public Health
    Reports 1896-1970*, 1924: p. 655-
    663.

Chapter 13

Allen, Robert W., and A. Walter Ecklund. "Botulism in North Dakota: Report of Outbreak of Thirteen Fatal Cases." *Journal of the American Medical Association*, vol. 99, no. 7, 1932, pp. 557-559.

The Bismarck Tribune. Bismarck, North Dakota, 10 Feb. 1931, p. 1.

C. Madsen. Bebeanna Greevers Chapiewski photo on FamilySearch, www.familysearch.org/tree /person/sources/KN1R-GZ8.

The Fargo Forum, Daily Republican, and Moorhead Daily News. 2 Feb. 1931.

Grafton News and Times, Grafton, North Dakota, 11 Feb. 1931.

Grand Forks Herald, Grand Forks, North Dakota, 3 Feb. 1931, p. 2; 5 Feb. 1931, p.1.

Grand Forks Herald, Grafton, North Dakota, 10 February, 1931.

McDonough, Stephen L. The Golden Ounce: A Century of Public Health in North Dakota. 1989.

Morning Pioneer. Mandan, North Dakota, 2 Feb. 1931, p. 7; 9 Feb. 1931, p. 1, p. 9;

Photo credit: Lisa Oby, Hein Family Photos, 29 Nov. 2024

The Walsh County Record. Grafton, North Dakota, 5 Feb. 1931, p. 1

Photos on book cover:

Physician photos courtesy of the National Library of Medicine

Family group eating Christmas lunch, Queensland, 1918
Courtesy of Redcliffe Museum Photographic Collection, Morten Bay Regional Libraries